# BREAKING FREE FROM

# CHEMICAL RELIGION

## AND FINDING YOUR WAY BACK TO HEALTH

DRS. DAVID AND KIMBERLY ERB, DC

# DISCLAIMER

Although the publisher and the authors have made every effort to ensure that the information in this book was correct at press time and while this publication is designed to provide accurate information in regard to the subject matter covered, the publisher and the authors assume no responsibility for errors, inaccuracies, omissions, or any other inconsistencies herein and hereby disclaim any liability to any party for any loss, damage, or disruption caused by errors or omissions, whether such errors or omissions result from negligence, accident, or any other cause. The views expressed by the testimonials do not necessarily represent those of the publisher and the authors.

# ENDORSEMENTS

"Breaking Free from the Chemical Religion is a bold contribution to the natural healthcare community and anyone who thinks outside the medical paradigm. In its pages, Drs. David and Kimberly provide readers a Biblical perspective on wellness that is sure to draw attention and inspire a movement towards health freedom."

> **-Jordan Rubin is America's Biblical Health Coach and one of the most respected natural health experts. He's the founder of Garden of Life and Ancient Nutrition. He is the New York Times bestselling author of The Maker's Diet and has written over twenty additional titles, including Patient Heal Thyself.**

"Drs. David and Kimberly have been working by my side to bring true healing to healthcare. Over the last 20 years they've become trusted friends. In today's environment, it's hard to know who to believe. We need more truth … Chemical Religion certainly exposes truth."

> **-Dr. Greg Loman is a New York Times best-selling author for his book *One Minute Wellness*, Co-Founder of MaxLiving and the co-creator of the guiding principles of MaxLiving and the 5 Essentials.**

"David and Kimberly Erb have exuded a passion for health and truth that has impacted our lives and many in Africa since 2006 when we first met!

Their pursuit of truth in the area of health and in their faith in the Creator who made the body to heal the body, has only intensified as the onslaught of toxic medicine has increased!

Through their research and years of experience, hundreds of people have found permanent healing solutions outside of the politicized and weaponized Big Pharma industry!

We have heard many testimonies of healing and restoration that have transpired because of the research and teaching by the Erb's. You will discover some of these in *Chemical Religion*!

Our hope is that as more and more genuine scientists and researchers look into the way that God created man, there will be a wave of health advocates who will follow the Erb's groundbreaking lead!"

> -**Tom Deuschle is a pastor, business leader, and an established author. He has published** *Building People Building Dreams, Surgical Prayer,* **and** *First Fruits.* **For over 40 years Pastor Tom has led a church planting movement throughout Africa, Europe, North America, and Asia. His wife, Bonnie is a musician, songwriter, gospel artist, international speaker, health and wellness advocate, and co-founder and pastor of Celebration Ministries International. She is also the author of** *The Great Connection.* **The power couple live in Zimbabwe, Africa.**

"Chemical Religion is well cited, hits hard, and serves as a wakeup call. Read it with an open mind and you'll question many aspects of our current symptom-based healthcare system that has failed much of the public. We all must stop putting our faith in habitual offender corporations that have consistently shown to value profits over human lives.

What I like about this book is that it also shares powerful personal stories and simple steps that allow you to take control of your health once and for all."

-**Matthew Loop Author of** *Social Media Made Me Rich* **&** *Cracking the Cancer Code*

"In a time when people are lost and confused about so many things; it's refreshing to see Christian Doctors take a stand to speak truth. Dr. David Erb and his wife, Dr. Kimberly Erb are exceptional in their field, but this only scratches the surface of who they are. They have a heart for people and a love for God that extends far beyond their clinic and community. Not only can you trust them to provide the facts you need, but more importantly they are grounded in God's word."

-**Dr. Rosie Gallegos Main, DC Author of Amazon Best Selling recipe book** *Dr. Rosie's MexiKeto Kitchen* **Contributing Author of** *Christian Living* **magazine**

"Finally, some good news! David and Kimberly Erb practice what they preach! Readers will discover their genuine desire and wisdom in helping others get and stay, healthy —minus the heartache of toxic, and pricy synthetic drugs and unnecessary surgeries. This book is compelling as well as eye-opening! I wholeheartedly recommend *Chemical Religion* to those hopeful for a more God given path to wellness."

-**Tracy Levinson, Bestselling author of** *Unashamed - Candid Conversations about Dating, Love, Nakedness, & Faith tracylevinson.com*

"Drs. David and Kimberly have always excelled clinically and this book will continue to amplify their message that the body is self-healing and needs no interference above all else. What a wonderful book teaching people simple truths on how to reclaim their health!"

-Dr. Nathan Thompson, DC Author of *Transformation 28*

"We have a major health care crisis that is fueled by the philosophy that there is a pill for every illness. Most people have little faith in their body's own innate ability to heal and repair. This book, *Chemical Religion*, will help awaken our society to the broken model of health care and give you actionable steps to improve your health and live out your God given potential! I highly recommend it!"

**-Dr. David Jockers DNM, DC, MS Best Selling Author of *The Fasting Transformation* and *The Keto Metabolic Breakthrough***

"Once you open *Chemical Religion* you won't be able to put it down! The authors have brilliantly summarized the fallacies and bureaucracy of modern medicine and the pharmacological spell that has been cast over the people of the world.

What I like about this book is that it's written in a way you can understand yet delivers 100% fact backed with science and references. If you are looking for a holistic and natural answer to your health problems – you will find it within the chapters.

This could, quite possibly, begin the ushering in of a new health care system - one that honors God and respects the sanctity of innate healing from within."

**-Dr. Aaron Ernst, DC, LM, PSCD and founder of the popular radio broadcast AskDrErnst.com**

"Dr. David and Dr. Kimberly through their own life experiences, hardships and traumas have become a dynamic force that is resilient and unstoppable not only for the Chiropractic and medical community but also for the Kingdom of God.

As a cancer overcomer by natural means, I know personally the impact the Erbs have had on my life as chiropractors and as my friends.

I have personally watched them give everything they have and steward the gifts God has given them to bring truth, hope and healing to a world that is in fear, pain and full of sickness.

Chemical Religion is a must read and a must have reference full of hope filled pages that are needed for this generation and beyond to continue to move forward and thrive into a true health filled way of life."

**-Andrea Thompson Integrative Health Practitioner and Author of *How I Beat Cancer***

"Drs. David and Kimberly Erb have been getting results for patients that are amazing. The field of health needs new voices like this. I've been waiting for years to read this book and am excited it has finally come out."

**-Dr. Lance Wallnau of Lance Learning Group in Dallas, Texas**

# ACKNOWLEDGMENTS

I want to dedicate this book to my dad. Carl Pinson, what the enemy meant for evil the Lord has used to make me the woman I am. Your life impacted me and now your death is impacting the world with truth and healing. It wasn't all in your head.

Thank you, Drs. Anna and Brian Loranger for introducing me to the Principle of Chiropractic. And to Dr. Randy Johns for teaching my husband true chiropractic care that saved his life. Your impact is recognized through all the patients' lives who come into our offices looking for the hope you gave us.

Thank you, Drs. Greg and Maryella for being the best of friends. As the co-founders of MaxLiving you are on the frontlines carrying this mission to the world.

Pastors Tom and Bonnie Deuschle you believed in us and partnered with us to bring a Health Center to Zimbabwe, Africa. I'll always treasure the miracles we saw together there.

Thank you, Lance Wallnau for planting the seed for this book prophetically that night all those years ago. God spoke powerfully through you and this book is evidence of His faithfulness.

Thank you, Rebecca Gates for accepting the arduous journey of putting what God deposited inside us down on paper and birthing it.

Pastor Tracy Eckert we admire and are grateful to you for fearlessly bringing us into your church to speak the unfiltered truth during a time when everyone else seemed to be silenced.

To our team - our tribe who work tirelessly to love and care for our patients - thank you for supporting us in this massive mission that the Lord has us on together.

Zac, Zoey and Zenee, we love you so much and are proud of the way that you all have gone against the grain and have made unpopular choices that your peers and teachers often criticized you for. You have made sacrifices your whole lives for the gospel of true health and healing. This message isn't just your parents' mission. Each of you have taken up the mantle from your earliest school years and continue now to find ways for your voice to be heard. You are growing more zealous than us if that's even possible.

"Son of man, I have made you a watchman for the house of Israel; therefore hear a word from My mouth, and give them warning from Me:" Ezekiel 3:17.

This book is the reflection of what God has opened our eyes to see and warn His people. He has made us watchman and we have to be obedient to that calling.

Thank you, Heavenly Father for entrusting us with such an honor.

# CONTENTS

# FOREWORD

I've been in ministry for fifteen years. As the senior pastor of Storehouse Church, I am careful to prayerfully consider those with whom I would set before my congregation. I have known Drs. David and Kimberly Erb for several years and have benefited tremendously from their knowledge of healing the human body. That's why I often bring them in to share truth with my congregation. Their influence within my church and my own family has made a healthful impact for which I am forever grateful. They have a message that needs to be heard by the body of Christ.

First, they love Jesus and preach the gospel not just to their patients but through what they believe about God's creation, the human body. They believe God's most perfect and precious creation - man, can heal if set free from the earthly system of chemical trauma. They love their patients really well and have incredible compassion. They serve tirelessly to see people free and fully alive, both spiritually and physically. They have patients that come to see them from all over the world.

They are incredibly gifted Chiropractors but so much more. When I first came into their office, I just thought I was going to get an adjustment for my shoulder pain. Instead what I got was a new family who helped me to heal and learn a new way to live healthy in our very complex world that is trying to kill us. Every time I hear them speak on the subject of health or vaccines, I am blown away by the level of detailed research. They both have photographic memories and remember the detailed statistics of everything they study. They are passionate about seeing people healed and physically free from pain and suffering. They have always been on the cutting edge of researching how to maximize health and minimize the damage from environmental substances, pharmaceutical poisoning and processed foods.

When I first began to learn from them, I was in denial. Then as I implemented their protocols, my energy and stamina returned and my brain fog and body pain left. I felt healthy for the first time in ten years. They have taught me a new way to cook, shop, and eat. I know about different ingredients in foods that maximize my health. I am working out and running again with no pain. I have personally brought at least one hundred people through their doors. That is how impacted I have been by their lives and protocols of health.

The Erb's are brilliant and have such a grasp on how the body processes different foods for healing and chemicals that harm. They take physiological facts and break them down so that anyone can be empowered by the truth of the body's functionality as designed by God. What they share in this book will change your outlook and understanding of how to care for your body and what to avoid to initiate healing.

Drs. David and Kimberly Erb are also incredibly knowledgeable about the "industry" of pharmaceuticals and how harmful their products are to humanity. In this book, they share what they have spent years researching and putting into practice resulting in people being set free from sickness and meds.

This is a compelling book that you will not be able to put down. It will wake you up and activate your personal responsibility in your journey towards health and wholeness, free from poisons and drugs in our food and medical system. I highly and joyfully recommend *Chemical Religion*.

**Tracy Eckert is the senior pastor of Storehouse Church and an intercessor at Dallas House of Prayer in Texas. She is also the author of *God's End-Time Temple*.**

# PREFACE

*David:*

We fell in love the first night we met. Moving together in beautiful harmony, Kimberly seemed to anticipate our next step together while still allowing me to lead her on the dance floor. I'll never forget how much fun we had together that night. *One step, two step* – these were the first we took together in unison, but they were only a foreshadowing of the steps God had planned for us to take together. After 24 years, Kimberly still moves beside me with that same anticipation for our next steps together, but we soon realized the one ordering our steps has always been God.

*Kimberly:*

I was 16 years old when I was pulled out of class and told that my dad had been in a car accident. I remember passing the scene on my way to the hospital and seeing the wreckage. It was bad. I didn't know what I was facing. I had always been "Daddy's little girl." We would go hunting together. He taught me to dance, and when he wasn't dancing with my mom, he was dancing with me. He was so full of life and fun. But upon arriving the hospital and seeing him lying on the gurney in pain made me wonder if things would ever be the same again.

After one week in the hospital the doctors declared Dad recovered and sent him home, but his pain left with him and continued to torment him. We didn't know what else to do, so we kept returning to the medical professionals hoping for answers and praying for a cure. After three and a half weeks of desperate persistence, they told us that it was all in my dad's head and recommended he see a psychiatrist. We obeyed the doctor's orders without question.

The psychiatrist was quick to prescribe the latest breakthrough in psychiatric medicine at the time, making my dad like a guinea pig for the new drug Prozac's side-effects. We saw the changes in him immediately. He couldn't remember how to do basic things. He became paranoid and angry, imagining that people were talking about him. When he was on these drugs he was not the same person.

My father was an avid hunter. He taught me about guns and the kinds of ammunition to use when killing an animal, so it doesn't suffer. He had a strong respect for human life, so he was careful to teach me about gun safety. But a week and a half after my dad began taking the mind-altering drug, he did something he never would've done in his right mind.

My Daddy was strong, but the dark voice inside his head was stronger. He waited until I left for gymnastics camp and my mom left for work before going into the garage to obey the pill's command. Manipulating a shot gun so that he would be able to pull the trigger on himself, Dad filled it with the kind of bullet that would cause terrible suffering and a slow death. He took his own life.

When my dad was suffering, we turned to the only hope we knew. We just did what the medical doctors told us to do, and my dad shot himself. Years later the black box warnings came out about the risks of suicide when taking Prozac and other antidepressants (SSRI's). If only we had known better. If only there had been other options presented to us, maybe my daddy would've been waiting up for me the night I fell in love with the man who danced with me the way my dad danced with my mom. Maybe he would've been there to walk me down the aisle and to sway with me on my wedding day one last time as his little girl.

After all that I had been through in watching my dad suffer after his injury then losing him to a medically induced mental illness, I was determined to spend my life finding answers. I wanted answers, to understand how this could have happened to me, but I also wanted to spend my life honoring my dad's memory and providing hope for others who were suffering the way he had. I never want another little girl to have to go through what I went through. David and I were married, but my dad wasn't there to walk me down the aisle.

## David:

We thought we were living happily ever after. Kimberly and I started a family. We had plans for our future together. That's why I didn't want to admit to her or to myself that something wasn't right. I was tired, fatigued and depressed. I was sick and hurting all the time even though I looked like a picture of health by any doctor's standard. After a year of suffering every day, I just got used to waking up that way.

One day my family was playing volleyball and I couldn't hide it anymore. My wife watched me pass out and hit the ground. I know she must've been so scared. When I came to, I had to face the truth, and I agreed to see a cardiologist.

The doctor entered the room with my test results. He said, "your heart is dying in your chest." After that I couldn't really hear anything else besides the pounding in my chest as if it were trying to keep pace with my own racing thoughts.

The blood drained from my face and in shock I locked eyes with my wife, inwardly begging her to tell me this wasn't real. As the doctor continued to give me my prognosis, I kept thinking, "This isn't happening." The future he was offering me was surgery and meds for the rest of my life—and an inactive lifestyle void of the physical activities I loved.

The medical doctors couldn't offer us hope for a cure. They didn't know what had been causing the pain in Kimberly's father nor what was causing the demise in my heart. The only options they could give us involved drugs and surgery that would come with a whole new set of debilitations, as my father-in-law had experienced. Their well-meaning answers would not make the pain go away. They would not allow true healing and recovery to resume and I wasn't willing to sacrifice my life to save it. Surgery was not an option for me, but I believed in the Great Physician, the One who could give me hope. The One who created my body knew how to heal it and he had the answers for me. It was another step I took with my wife in our dance together. Now we were in sync, both searching for the answers that could save me while also bringing meaning to her dad's death, *if* we could discover how to help others.

The day I was led to a chiropractor who understood subluxation is the day my life changed. Doctor Randy Johns cared enough to agree to meet me halfway at a restaurant where he spent seven hours going over the Principle of Chiropractic with me. Kimberly and I were already chiropractors, but we had never been taught the things Dr. Randy was sharing. I left that restaurant with more than a full stomach. I left with my purpose, my calling and answers to my healing. I had hope again and I could already feel the depression lifting.

This doctor took chiropractic to a whole new level and showed me how to discover the cause of the symptoms I was experiencing. I was like most people who believe they're healthy until symptoms occur or a diagnosis is given. I soon learned that *health starts at function.* My wife became my chiropractor, having learned from Dr. Johns. She was able to take some x-rays and locate what was interfering with my health. She began to correct my spine through Advanced Spinal Corrective adjustments and rehabilitation. After only one month I was symptom-free and 18 months later my spine was fully corrected. And my heart was healed.

I went back to the cardiologist to confirm what I already knew. After my examination he looked at me suspiciously and said, "It looks like you have a new heart."

My wife and I decided to change the course of our lives so that we can change the course of others' lives as well. We have made it our mission to continue to educate ourselves so that we can educate our patients. Now, as doctors who correct the spine, we have become experts in offering hope and healing to our patients. We've been on the other side. I know what it feels like to be sick, to be afraid and I can tell you, it feels amazing to feel good again. I'll never take my health for granted or expect it to simply always be there.

My experience has made me an unstoppable force, working to make sure every human being lives their life to its greatest potential. I hope in writing this book and by presenting the answers and hard truths that very few are talking about we can prevent more people from facing the same wake-up call I experienced. I hope we can bring deliverance from the fears spread in a culture that looks solely to the medical and pharmaceutical industry for cures they can't provide.

### *Kimberly:*

David and I have dedicated our lives to finding the cause of our patients' symptoms, those things that are robbing them of a life more abundant, and then correcting the issue so their body can heal itself the way God created it to. This is why I get up in the morning. Every day I am face-to-face with families who are scared and hurting just like mine was. But I get to listen to them and tell them "This isn't just in your head. Let me show you what is causing your troubles and we will bring healing to it together. You are not alone." And every time I see their hope restored, I feel my dad's pride for the impact that his life has made.

Don't become a guinea pig for pharmaceutical companies. Follow us to hope.

# CHAPTER 1
# HAVE YOU BEEN
# INDOCTRINATED?

" For your merchants were the greatest in the world, and you deceived the nations with your sorceries [*pharmakeia*]." Revelation 18:23b NLT

Western civilization boasts the greatest healthcare in history, which is lucky I suppose, since so many people are diagnosed with something. Young or old, it seems that everyone is getting sick, and those who aren't are scared they'll be next. The National Heart Association would say that the number one cause of death is heart disease. The American Cancer Society reports deaths in terrifying numbers as well, but the pharmaceutical industry has a dirty little secret they're keeping from you, a secret so dark it could ruin the trust they have spent hundreds of millions of dollars to establish, thus keeping you in their pockets and under their control.

Their fear tactics lure you back to them for more of whatever they're producing. Their message of salvation is preached from radio, television, billboards and social media. Your friends, your family, your school and your healthcare providers are evangelists for the doctrine Big Pharma is spreading. And, whether you realize it or not, you're being indoctrinated into their Chemical Religion.

Their secret? *The number one cause of death in the United States isn't disease, it's the medicine they teach the medical doctors to prescribe.* Like a priest serving wafers of atonement for sins, the medical profession expects you to open wide for the pills they are serving.

Pharmaceutical companies will do just about anything to keep you from escaping their grips. When indoctrination doesn't work, they will use scare tactics and control. Refuse their vaccines and your child will not be allowed to go to school. If your student doesn't go to school, you'll find yourself in truancy court.

Many children whose parents have refused the prescribed treatments have been taken from their family and forced into compliance by Child Protective Services. At least one family experienced a SWAT team showing up to their home with CPS. It was a terrifying experience for the family, and it made a big statement to anyone watching. Comply or else.

I remember being in the most vulnerable position, laying on a table about to deliver my youngest daughter. My doctor, with scalpel in hand, was about to cut me open for my caesarean section when a nurse walked in carrying my file. She pointed out my choice to refuse the use of Ilotycin. The antibiotic is put in a newborn's eyes to prevent the risk of exposure to Chlamydia and Gonorrhea as the baby enters the birth canal. It causes burning and stinging to our precious little bundles as we welcome them into the world for the first time. Besides the fact I didn't have any STD's, my baby wasn't even being delivered vaginally! The nurse piously announced that she would be calling CPS if I refused her potion. The peaceful atmosphere I had created with beautiful music playing in the background for my birth experience was immediately replaced with fear and anxiety.

This example—at the moment of birth, is just the beginning of their plans. Money is not made from people who ask too many questions and think for themselves. Stories like mine terrorize us into submission to their doctrines. If they can't convince you, they'll scare you into believing you won't survive without them. If that doesn't work, they'll use the power they have with the government to force you into compliance. Our nation's rights are slowly being revoked because many of us are too scared or indoctrinated to rise up.

Since forcing their products upon us this $1.2 trillion industry has taken credit for the demise of many diseases, while they ignore the rise of cancers and many other illnesses that have plagued us since they started poking us and mixing potions containing preservatives, lab altered viruses and bacteria; aluminum; mercury; formaldehyde; phenoxyethanol; gluteraldehyde; sodium borate; sodium chloride; sodium acetate; monosodium glutamate (MSG); hydrochloric acid; hydrogen peroxide; lactose; gelatin; yeast protein; egg albumin; bovine and human serum albumin; antibiotics; phenol (carbolic acid), borax (ant killer), ethylene glycol (antifreeze), dye, acetone (nail polish remover), latex, glycerol, polysorbate 80/20, sorbitol and other unidentified contaminants. Children are being injected with some of the most lethal poisons known, but is it worth the risk?

Don't be fooled: 85% of medicine is based on tradition rather than science. This faith-based cult's practices can only attribute 2% of its cures to its medicine, the other 98% are placebo effect. "Beware lest anyone cheat you through philosophies and empty deceit, according to the basic principles of the world, and not according to Christ." Colossians 2:8 NKJV.

### Are Vaccines Really to Thank for the End of Diseases?

It's true, the mortality rate for many diseases have dramatically decreased. I used to buy into the marketing that modern medicine was to thank for the decline until I dug a little deeper. Scarlet fever, diphtheria, whooping cough (also known as pertussis) and measles declined by 90% between 1860 and

1965, which was before the introduction of antibiotics and widespread immunizations.

From 1923-1953, before the polio vaccine was introduced, its death rate in the U.S. had already declined on its own by 47% and in the UK by 55%. However, the number of cases of polio peaked immediately after the vaccine came out and then continued its downward slide like the others. Those numbers don't add up to the message Big Pharma is preaching.

The evidence indicates that advancements in our living conditions such as clean water and running water with indoor plumbing, less crowding and an overall higher standard of living made a huge impact on the health of our nation and other developed nations. Even today you can see the difference in the wellness of the United States in contrast to countries without such advancements. (However, this seems to be changing as we continue to put our faith in the Chemical Religion and bite into the marketing the food industry is serving.)

In the 1800's towns were over-populated, and plumbing was virtually non-existent. The raw sewage from people and animals drained into the drinking water. Trash piled up everywhere, which became a breeding home and in turn caused massive rat infestations. One city reported over 700,000 rats! The government was calling on people to kill as many as they were able in an effort to stop the rodents from further destruction.

The over-worked families included children as young as four years old working 17-hour shifts. Child labor of the 1800's was like Nazi concentration camps, especially for those who never saw the light of day due to working in coal mines under dangerous circumstances. Tired, malnourished women were miscarrying their babies and exposing themselves to doctors who did not yet know the importance of washing their hands.

Food was scarce and the commercial food industry wanted to make money even if it meant selling meats and vegetables that were spoiled or rotten. But people were poor and desperate. Entire families were sleeping on the

Chapter 1 Have You Been Indoctrinated?

floors of one-room apartments that were actually closets in a house where multiple families paid rent. They ate what little they could get, which was most often bad food void of nutrients. They drank contaminated water. They wore their bodies down and they neglected sunlight and ventilation. They were ignorant of proper cleanliness and sanitization practices. Sickness was sure to come—and it stayed until the government took measures to clean up and set standards for humane business practices, including the enforcement of wholesome food sales.

During this same period the use of vaccinations continued to be passionately argued. Despite the declining numbers in mortality, medical scientists relentlessly experimented with the creation of vaccines while manipulating numbers to support their necessity, something they continue to do today. The use of vaccinations was dropping, so M.D.s were told to diagnose whooping cough rather than bronchitis, a cold, or other conditions having similar symptoms. Suddenly they were able to announce an "epidemic" of whooping cough. The profession gloated, "See, we told you so" but the actual numbers don't lie. After parents stopped pertussis vaccinations in the UK, the death rate from whooping cough was the lowest in recorded history.

Official returns from Germany show that between 1870 and 1885, one million vaccinated persons died from smallpox. Of 9,392 smallpox patients in London hospitals in 1871, 6,854 had been vaccinated with 17.5% of those ending in death. But Pharma still took credit for the declining numbers and twisted the evidence to serve their purposes.

Vaccinations have become an unquestionable part of our society. But maybe we need to start asking some questions, like why is there a growing number of new or expanding illnesses such as heart disease, autism, more cancers, SIDs, asthma, ADHD, brain inflammation (Encephalitis), erectile dysfunction, food and other allergies, dyslexia, Crohn's disease, ulcerative colitis and all kinds of auto immune diseases since the pharmaceutical companies have supposedly provided us with better health?

By law M.D.s must report vaccine injuries to the government's Vaccine Adverse Event Reporting System (VAERS), but according to the FDA only one in ten vaccine-injured children is ever reported. Many caring medical professionals find this alarming. "The number one place parents bring their kids in the event of a vaccine reaction is the E.R., and *as an E.R. nurse,* I have NEVER met anyone who filed one, despite seeing hundreds of cases of obvious vaccine-associated harm come through. What does that say about reported numbers?" – An ER nurse from Nurses Against Vaccines.

Doctors and nurses who have questioned the rituals of their industry have been shunned, cast out and even professionally ruined when they try to do what's right. Just like the rest of us, they're bullied into compliance and silenced by a greedy "higher power."

### In it for the Money or for the Cure?

Not-so coincidentally, the pharmaceutical companies are owned by powerful families who set up all medical schools to push medicine for their own profit. Aspiring medical doctors become indoctrinated at these schools. One doctor confessed she never had time to question what was being taught because the academic load was too intense, but over time she began to realize how much of what she had learned didn't make sense.

In the 1980's the pharmaceutical companies were sometimes held accountable with multiple lawsuits asserting their products were dangerous. The compensations they paid out cut into their profits, so they manipulated the government into believing that there would be a vaccine shortage that would threaten the health of our country if it didn't do something to protect their bottom line. That's when the National Vaccine Injury Compensation Program (VICP) was formed, and since the first claims were filed in 1989, more than $3 **billion** in compensation awards has been paid to petitioners. More than $120.4 million has been paid to cover attorneys' fees and other legal costs with taxpayers' money. Big Pharma has a sweet deal by charging outrageously for products that consumers are forced to buy and then charging us again to pay for their mistakes.

But those aren't the only questions we should be asking. Let's ask the medical doctors why there's a higher rate of chronic diseases in those who have been vaccinated?

## Do the Benefits Really Outweigh the Risks?

The vaccine schedule has dramatically changed from when I was a child, receiving only six vaccines. Now it's up to 49 doses by the 1st grade! Every year pharmaceutical companies are coming up with more vaccines and drugs. By the time a child is six months old it is injected with 48 vaccines; at 18 months the number is 70; and at 4-6 years *at least* 89 doses of toxin-containing shots are to have been injected into your children! We wouldn't let our babies near some of these ingredients on the playground, but we take them in for their wellness check-up and hold their little legs down while they cry out in fear and pain begging us to protect them from the fateful needles.

Many parents have come through our office baring the regret of not having asked the questions, of going with the flow and now living with a child suffering from the effects of a vaccine. They struggle to forgive themselves because every day is a reminder of their misguided trust in the Chemical Religion. These parents know without a doubt the cause of their child's sickness in the same way any other parent can pinpoint what's going on with their kids, but they get zero validation or help from the injecting doctors. What's even more disheartening are the other parents who venomously criticize our patients when they dare to speak out and share their stories in hopes of saving others from similar experiences.

Whenever vaccination criticism surfaces, the media will interview some health department official or M.D. who will repeat the mantra: "Sure, vaccines have some slight chance of causing damage, but [*repeat after me*] 'the benefits far outweigh the risks.'" The only problem with that statement is that it has never been proven. No one knows what the chances are that your child may be hurt or killed by a vaccine. In order to do a risk-benefit analysis we need to know how many children are being hurt. We don't know because M.D.s and health officials aren't reporting vaccine injuries. We're being forced to inject chemicals into our children and have no idea if it's even safe! Are you beginning to see how blind faith in the Chemical Religion has caused such destruction?

My husband and I have been asking the questions for a long time now. We keep asking the questions even though we've already discovered the answers, because we want to invoke change. We want to get people thinking for themselves. We have gathered more studies and stats than we could ever put in this book, but here are just a few to prove how the medical industry has been lying to you, and hopefully entice you into further research on your own. We're living in an age where it's imperative that we stay informed.

- Immunized children: 23.1% had asthma, and 30% had other allergic illnesses vs. non-immunized children, where 0% had asthma or other allergic illness.

- Pertussis vaccination and asthma: 10.69% of children immunized (with pertussis) got asthma.

- 62 studies from 30 worldwide laboratories link the polio vaccine to brain tumors, bone cancers, lung lining cancers and leukemia.

- The rates of the cancers listed above have gone up dramatically in the last 30 years.

- Pediatric cancer has been rising 1% a year since 1974 and is the second-leading cause of death in children (after accidental injuries).

- Leukemia and brain tumors are the most common childhood malignancies, showing a 35% rise in pediatric brain cancer between 1973 and 1994.

Between mid 1999 and 2004 there were 128,035 adverse reactions reported to the VAERS, which may represent between 1.28 – 12.8 million of the actual vaccine-associated adverse reactions. Maybe if it isn't your child you're putting at risk it's easy to say, "the benefits far outweigh the risks," but with these numbers alone, I have to disagree with Big Pharma's mantra.

Laurie Forbes, MD, Medical Director of the Metropolitan Cancer Hospital in London says, "I am convinced that the increase of cancer is due to vaccination." Have we traded mumps and measles for cancer and leukemia? What about autoimmune diseases? Why is it that 24 million Americans have some sort of autoimmune disease when just prior to 1989 the chronic disease rate was only 12.8%, verses 54% one year later?

I see people flocking to the slaughter with scales on their eyes and it feels so lonely to have the answers, only to be ignored. Fear has deafened them to the solutions that could save them. That's exactly what it feels like for us as practitioners who have been freed from the Chemical Religion. Patients come into our office and we're able to tell them the truth that gives them hope, but they have been so indoctrinated to believe they'll die if they don't do what the medical doctors advise. They return to join the droves looking for a diagnosis and will be lucky if they don't become another statistic.

If our healthcare is so exceptional than why is our life expectancy declining? It's certainly not for the lack of medicine, since the vast majority of pharmaceuticals are consumed in the U.S. It seems that our fears are misguided. Instead of running *to* the medical doctors who are controlled by a greedy industry forcing harmful medications on patients, maybe you should be running away from them. Maybe you should be breaking free from their Chemical Religion.

There is hope down a straight and narrow road where few gather, but those who are brave enough tread upon it are thriving. Follow us to hope and healing.

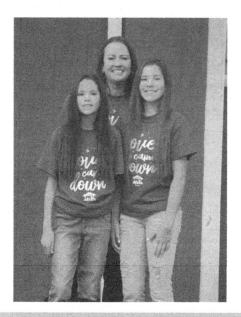

My family started going to Erb Family Wellness in 2006. We were all on anti-depressants and anti-anxiety meds. We were in a bad way. I came to them with a lot of back pain. I had had a procedure 10 years earlier to relieve the pain, but it never worked. I was in pain all the time.

Since being under the care of the Erbs, my family and I were able to get off the medications and my back pain is significantly better.

We learned so much from Erb Family Wellness and have seen how what they teach works. That's why when my grandmother was diagnosed with breast cancer, we wanted to tell her the good news of hope. Sadly, when we tried to talk to her about true health that we were experiencing from the Erbs, we were laughed out of the house for thinking that healing could come outside of a medical hospital. It was so hard for us to watch my grandmother suffer through the chemotherapy and eventually pass away. But we were very thankful to get better information from Dr. David for our own health.

When I had my girls, I was thankful Dr. David could refer me to a birthing center. I was also thankful for the knowledge that in the state of Texas, I had the choice whether to vaccinate my children or not. My girls have never had meds, fast food or soda. That wasn't a problem until public school. Teachers would laugh at my kids for eating radishes for school snacks. They loved nutritious foods. Their appetites had not been spoiled by toxic packaged foods.

I don't know what we would do without Dr. David. We love seeing him every week and to be able to text him anytime we need him, have questions, or just need prayer. I feel like we have someone on our side. If we were to have to go to the ER for some reason, he would be there for us. – Candi Creaser

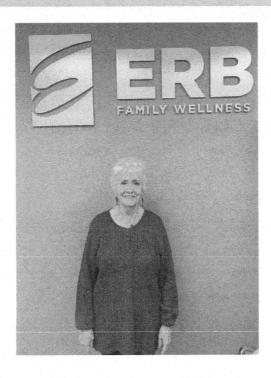

I've been going to Erb Family Wellness for a little under 20 years. In the beginning I followed their most advanced diet protocol and it worked well to lose weight and feel better. But when my husband died, I started eating bad again.

I started feeling really bad in 2021. My OBGYN doctor told me I had a large fibroid and I needed surgery. After my surgery at the end of February, I was told that cancer was not detected. But later a pathologist determined that cancer was found deep within the fibroid. My doctor wanted me to do chemotherapy. She kept saying, "Well, just to be safe." But it didn't feel right that the oncology was connected to the gynecology in this office. It seemed like a conflict of interest. What Dr. Erb had taught me about health rang in my head.

As I weighed out my options, I talked to a couple of the gynecologist's patients my age who had survived the chemo. I also talked to the gynecologist's dietician who was saying all the opposite things that Dr. Erb had taught me about nutrition. It was cause for concern when I considered putting myself under the care of the doctor who had hired him to help her patients.

While in the office, I noticed some of the chemo patients who were bluish gray, and I knew I couldn't do that to myself. When I respectably told my doctor my decision, she turned around and with the most horribly angry face said, "Well I'm not the one who only has six months to live!" I felt like I was looking evil in the face.

By the end of March, I submitted myself to the care of Erb Family Wellness. I threw myself into eating healthy and getting adjusted. Dr. Kimberly put me on a protocol to get the toxins out of my body. I also went into the hyperbaric chamber.

It's been a long road, but I am feeling so much better. I started walking and jogging intervals. I'm increasing the jogging and will soon increase the distance. I'm even starting to lift weights at 73 years old.

I'm past the six-month marker and I'm not dead yet. The main point I would like to make is for people to wake up and listen to Dr. David and Dr. Kimberly. I wasted so many years and didn't do what the Erbs said to do. Maybe if I had, I would not have ended up with a diagnosis that I could've avoided. – Patty Mount

# CHAPTER 2
# FORBIDDEN FRUIT: HAVE YOU HAD YOUR FILL?

"The fruit will be good food, and the leaves will be used for healing."

Ezekiel 47:12b GWT

From the beginning of creation man has been enticed by forbidden fruit. God provided a garden full of wholesome goodness for man to eat, but the serpent suggested the fruit from the tree God forbade offered something more. Satan strategically planted a seed that, once consumed, grew into a harvest of evil and death.

We read the story and wonder how Adam and Eve could've bitten into such a lie, then we sit mesmerized by advertising that appeals to our lusts for faster, easier, and healthier—all without sacrifice. We're no less deceived by marketing today than the first couple in the garden were by the snake's propaganda. From the beginning he had an agenda to steal from us, to kill us and to destroy us. The saddest part is that we're letting him.

## From Forbidden Fruit to Medicalization

Medicalization started in the Garden when the serpent suggested that God had created man with lack. The sly snake suggested that God was keeping the couple from reaching their highest potential and offered the forbidden fruit as a cure. Medicalization is the process by which human conditions and problems come to be defined and treated as medical conditions, thus becoming the subject of medical study, diagnosis, prevention or treatment. Big Pharma, the food industry and Big Business seem to have worked together to create a problem for which Chemical Religion can sell a solution.

The food industry entices us with toxic and nutrient-deficient choices, making us sick and in search of a doctor to prescribe something. We want them to prophecy that we're going to be okay as long as we do everything they command. We take the medicine made by the pharmaceutical company, though it's not meant to cure anything, but rather it masks our symptoms while creating *new* symptoms for which we will need *another* pill. We keep buying into the lie.

### Leaving the Garden for a Lie

"95% of all cancer is due to diet and the accumulation of toxins."

- University of Columbia School of Public Health

God created a whole garden of goodness for mankind to enjoy. This garden brings nourishment to our bodies, but somewhere along the line we deviated from His plan. The Western Diet consumed by most of us in the U.S. is made of poor-quality foods having a shelf life that will outlast your dog. Besides refined grains, the highly addictive ingredient sugar is found in everything from granola bars to salad dressing. We don't even realize how addicted we are to this sweet substance. It is strategically snuck into our food under a variety of different names to keep us coming back for another fix. Watch out for these sugar aliases:

- Corn sweetener
- Corn syrup
- Dextrose fructose
- Fruit juice concentrates
- Glucose
- Maltose
- Invert sugar
- Lactose
- High-fructose corn syrup
- Raw sugar
- Sucrose
- Sugar syrup
- Cane crystals
- Cane sugar
- Crystalline fructose
- Evaporated cane juice
- Corn syrup solids
- Malt syrup

The average person unknowingly consumes 57 pounds of added sugar a year —and we wonder why cancer, heart disease and diabetes continue to rise. The food industry and Big Pharma aren't willing to be honest about the effects of sugar on our health. Even the FDA seems suspicious, slapping all kinds of discrediting warnings on naturally grown supplemental products known to truly heal ailments, while backing the substance proven to be as addictive and harmful as cocaine. It's not too difficult to figure out who is profiting from our dependence on this sweet, white substance.

## What Changed?

In 1955 President Dwight Eisenhower suffered a heart attack, which put sugar in the spotlight. The U.S. and England each sought counsel from medical scientists. One doctor argued that a diet high in sugar was to blame for Eisenhower's heart disease while the other countered that a diet rich in fat was the culprit. Sugar won the battle, making fat the enemy. Our food industry's marketing changed. More sugars were added to compensate for the fats that were being removed. This "low-fat" boasting nonsense has continued for years!

In 1990, Dr. Walter Willett of Harvard University found that by evaluating the best studies to date, no correlation existed between saturated fat intake and the risk of heart disease. Further diet studies conducted in 1995 and 1997 revealed similar results, yet people keep looking for the "fat free" labels while loading up on sugar.

Globally, the sugar and sweetener market hit $97 billion in 2017. It's not easy combatting a superpower of that magnitude. It can afford the resources necessary to make the truth practically disappear. In the 70's the U.S. government began reviewing the safety of sugar, but the powers that be were quick to fight back. Taking tips from the tobacco industry, the sugar industry launched its own campaign. It paid scientists for junk studies and PR companies to make deceptive statements dispelling the public's fears. The bittersweet superpower knew that as long as there was not a consensus, people could believe what they wanted to believe. Parents could still feel good about giving their kids the sugary cereals they craved. Couples could continue to indulge in desserts after romantic dinners together. Life could go on, addicted in ignorant bliss.

Fortunately, there are still some medical professionals who aren't convinced by the food industry's lies. In a groundbreaking study, Dr. Kimber Stanhope PhD, MS, an Associate Project Scientist in the Department of Molecular Biosciences at the University of California, Davis disproved the old mantra, "a calorie, is a calorie, is a calorie." Her study proved that high fructose corn syrup consumption causes heart disease, diabetes and strokes. The evidence proving that proper nutrition and food is important way beyond just calories and obesity is overwhelming. For example, 22 almonds have the same number of calories as a Twinkie. It's common sense that consuming almonds is the healthier option.

Sugar is toxic and contains only empty calories, but products that boast about being "sugar-free" usually contain poisonous artificial sweeteners like aspartame. We'll explain more in the next chapter, but for now we suggest that you use Stevia and erythritol to replace sugar.

Trying to avoid fake, sugar-filled and chemically altered foods can make grocery shopping challenging. Avoiding the middle isles where the packaged foods are is best, but not always possible. In our shopping we make sure the food we bring home has these labels:

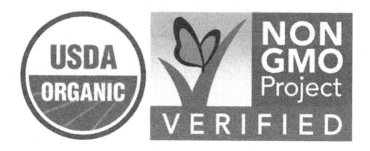

- **BPA-free** – Does not contain the industrial chemical BPA

- **Non-GMO** – Verifies it does not contain genetically modified organisms.

- **USDA Organic** – Organic products meeting the USDA requirements.
    - Produced without excluded methods, (*e.g.*, genetic engineering, ionizing radiation, or sewage sludge).
    - Produced using allowed substances.

When shopping for produce, the label is the number code listed on the attached sticker. Look for five-digit codes ending in the number nine.

Product Label Cheat:

4 Digit                                        → Conventional Grown.

5 Digit ends with '9'     → Organic.

5 Digit ends with '8'     → GMO Farmed.

## GMOs and Other Fake Foods

The dangers of genetically modified foods have been overlooked in the U.S., but in the U.K. they're mostly prohibited. In some starving countries GMO foods sound like the answer to their problem. In 2006 we went to Zimbabwe, Africa for the first time. We worked with a local church to begin educating people about how to care for their bodies with diet, exercise, spinal correction and maintenance. In just one week after our first clinic's grand opening, we had 1,500 new patients!

Kimberly and the kids traveled from the U.S. to Zimbabwe frequently over the next five years opening four more clinics and helping tens of thousands of patients change their lives. We were on a mission to change a nation that had been known for its suffering. More than 50 doctors and students had come to lend their support and join in the revolution. The impact we were making gave us a level of influence with government officials, or so we thought.

When we first started serving in Zimbabwe the people were used to consuming one meal a day of a corn-grits-like meal called *sadzu*. When the agricultural domain was told they could feed more starving people if they genetically modified the food, we pleaded with them to reconsider. To the country's detriment, our cautions were ignored changing the texture and appearance of the *sadzu* from the original dark, dense nutrient packed meal to a fluffy bowl of sugary, bleached, manmade potion.

In October of 2010 we took what we didn't know would be our last trip to what had become our second home. Instead of receiving support or gratitude from the African government for our work in its country, we were not welcomed back. Kicked out of the country and confused, we realized something: corrupt governments aren't afraid of sick citizens revolting against it. It would rather the people seek help from witch doctors than to grow stronger from the truth we were administering. It would rather give the people full bellies that lead to disease than protect them.

"There is a way that appears to be right, but in the end, it leads to death" Proverbs 14:12 NIV. Before Zimbabwe introduced GMOs to its food source, the main disease that was killing people was HIV. Now the diseases also include diabetes, digestive disease, heart disease and cancer. As soon as you compromise God's seed for fake food, you won't be able to measure the amount of disease.

GMOs also wreak havoc on intestinal health. With 85% of our immune system residing in our intestinal lining, it's no wonder that there is over-whelming evidence showing that these foods cause leaky gut syndrome, heightened food allergies, auto immune disease and a number of inflammatory health issues.

Glyphosate (found in Roundup and used on genetically modified plants) interferes with Cytochrome P450 (CYP), an enzyme necessary for the human body to detox and decrease aging. CYP is how the good bacteria in our digestive tract functions to process foods into necessary amino acids, hormones, neurotransmitters and many other components critical for good health. Glyphosate starts a chain reaction, starving the body from critical nutrient processes and inducing leaky gut.

Other research confirms that eating GM foods alters our genes, limiting our ability to burn sugar correctly, thus making us fatter. According to research from the University of California and Washington State University, GMO plants are sicker, requiring more pesticide and fertilizers to grow. The plants then offer very little nutrition and are covered in chemicals. Over time, some weeds have mutated to resist Roundup, requiring nearly four times their recommended activation rate to be effective. This increases the amount used all over the world each year.

## How Important is Gut Health?

One of the key functions of the gut is to break down food and absorb nutrients. Having healthy gut microbiome aids in digestion. Our intestinal microbiome plays an important role in normal gut function. They're the good soldiers fighting for our gut health in the same way that probiotics are the beneficial microorganisms that inhabit the gastrointestinal tract. They fight the invasion of bad bacteria and help you utilize your nutrition to create energy and vitamins.

The gut barrier acts as a divider between the bloodstream and the external environment to allow nutrients in and keep toxins, antigens and bad bacteria out. Our body cannot absorb nutrients properly when we have unhealthy or unbalanced microflora. Besides the GMOs and toxic chemicals sprayed on our produce, there are several other factors that contribute to our gastrointestinal ill health.

- Bacterial growth
- Sugar intake
- Alcohol intake
- Consumption of processed foods

- Eating on the go
- Pain medications
- Antibiotic use
- Antibiotic exposure through exposed meats and byproducts such as dairy

Antibiotics decrease the body's ability to absorb nutrients and inflammation, which causes mitochondria to break down. Our gut contains a community of microorganisms, known as "gut flora," which has both good and harmful bacteria. For optimal digestive and immune health, these bacteria should remain balanced with as much good and as little harmful bacteria as possible. An imbalance in this gut flora can affect the progression of diseases, including cancer, both directly and indirectly. Antibiotics kill not only the *bad* bacteria, but they kill the *good* bacteria as well, leaving the body more susceptible to catch the next thing to which it's exposed. If the gut is left unhealed, yeast issues, food sensitivities and autoimmune diseases can occur.

When these issues occur, we recommend detoxing and diet change. Detoxification aids in nutrient absorption by resetting our digestion process. One study illustrates that healthy gut microbes enhanced growth and corrected metabolic abnormalities in malnourished children, increasing their bone density and muscle. Dr. Kellyann Petrucci, states, "If you have a sick, inflamed gut, you'll experience anything from wrinkled skin, to weight gain, to autoimmune disorders, to depression."

### What Else is Making Us Sick?

Hazardous toxins that cause illness are everywhere. They are being marketed to us as necessary.

- 4 billion prescription drugs are ingested in the U.S. each year
- 70,000 chemicals are used commercially
- 3,000+ chemicals are added to our food supply
- 10,000+ chemicals are used in food processing, preserving and storage

The Environmental Protection Agency (EPA) estimates that our homes are now 5 to 100 times more toxic than outdoor air. Some say the EPA isn't doing much to protect us from harmful chemicals like Roundup and wonder about their continued stance on the argument for the product's carcinogenic concerns.

As we mentioned above, Roundup is the brand name of a glyphosate-based herbicide originally produced by Monsanto, then acquired by Bayer in

2018. Glyphosate is the most widely used herbicide in the United States. Monsanto developed and patented the glyphosate molecule in the 1970's and marketed it as Roundup from 1973. Some 300 million pounds of glyphosate are used on crops worldwide each year. Monsanto also created genetically modified plants to resist the effects of his herbicide. But is it all safe?

Gilles-Eric Seralini of the University of Caen and his colleagues said that rats fed genetically modified corn (or given water containing Roundup) at levels permitted in the United States died earlier than those on a standard diet. The animals on the genetically modified diet suffered mammary tumors as well as severe liver and kidney damage. The researchers said 50% of males and 70% of females died prematurely, compared with only 30% and 20% that were not given the contaminated meals or water.

Roundup has been linked to lymphatic cancers in agricultural laborers and gardeners and is facing thousands of lawsuits. Three cases have already earned the validation from juries with verdicts of $289 million, $80 million and $2 billion against Monsanto. A recent article reported that Bayer is close to agreeing to a settlement of $8-10 billion for Roundup's harmful effects. This all seems a bit incriminating. The fact that the company has lost multiple lawsuits and is willing to settle for an even greater loss, indicates that the amount of money lost isn't significant enough in comparison to the amount of money made. But there are countless others who have not been compensated for the effects of this evil product. This hit too close to home for me when my best friend's brother died in 2019 from brain cancer caused from his daily use of Roundup.

### But as Long as We Don't Use Roundup We Won't Be Exposed, Right?

Our youngest daughter was only three years old when her routine Metabolic Testing (See Chapter 13 for MT explanation) indicated cancer and toxicity markers caused by a pesticide spray. We were shocked and obviously concerned. We wondered how this could be since our home was chemical free.

I went to her preschool to acquire information about the kinds of cleaning products they used and discovered that the building had recently been treated with bug spray. Piecing together the clues I was able to determine that my daughter's risk for cancer came from her naptime, spent lying on the floor where the spray had been spread.

The increase in glyphosate use makes the chemical almost impossible to avoid, even for those who don't directly handle Roundup. Traces of glyphosate have been found in oatmeal, honey, wine and even baby food. Cheerios has over 11 parts per billion! Just to give you an idea of how outrageous these amounts are, independent research shows that probable harm to human health begins at really low levels of exposure – at .1 Many foods were found to have over 1,000 times this amount, well above what regulators throughout the world consider "safe".

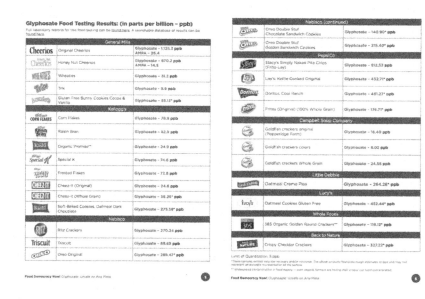

Glyphosate is now being used by some farmers in an 'off-label' fashion, as a pre-harvest desiccant (drying agent) on non-GMO food crops. Some farmers use glyphosate to force their crops to ripen early. If used in this way rather than as an herbicide the **non-GMO** label can still be used on the food even though it has been fully soaked in the hazardous liquid! It's becoming common for crops such as wheat, barley, oats and beans allowing farmers to get a faster harvest even in areas with a short growing season.

Even animals such as the ones we consume have been discovered to carry traces of glyphosate. Those of us who are trying to minimize our exposure by purchasing organic products are still at risk. The runoff from Roundup crops feed glyphosate into neighboring streams and rivers, from which our animal food supply drinks.

In a study conducted by the Detox Project, 93% of volunteer test participants had traces of glyphosate in their bodies. Even scarier, children reported higher percentages of the chemical on average. According to the Environmental Working Group (EWG), tests show 287 industrial chemicals were found in 10 newborn babies—with 180 of those being cancer-causing, 217 being toxic to the brain and nervous system and 208 causing birth defects or abnormal development. Our lust for faster, easier, healthier has come with great sacrifice.

Toxins are in cleaning products, detergents, cookware, personal care products, baby products; you name it! We're never going to escape chemicals, but we can minimize them if we stay educated. Check out our what-to-avoid list resource in the appendix. Study it and be empowered as the gatekeeper of your home.

## Why Isn't Our Government Protecting Us?

*"The officials* make a feast for enjoyment [instead of repairing what is broken], and serve wine to make life merry, and money
is the answer to everything"
Ecclesiastes 10:19 Amplified.

- The FDA has approved approximately 3,000 food additives, preservatives, and colorings.

- The average person ingests 150 pounds of additives every year.

- 90% or more of all U.S. grown corn, soybeans, canola and sugar beets are genetically modified, which means that virtually all processed food items contain at least one or more GMO ingredient.

There's a saying that was first popularized from a movie about Watergate in the 70's called *All the President's Men*: "Follow the money" to find the scandal. As Americans, we hear of other nations' corrupt governments, but are offended at the suggestion that our government could ever fall prey to the kind of greed it takes to so grossly misuse power. We can't forget the garden and the serpent's agenda. He will use even well-meaning people to accomplish his mission to destroy us. How much more might he use the greedy?

For example, with so much evidence against Roundup, how does the EPA refuse to proclaim the product a carcinogen? Why isn't the FDA putting stronger warning labels on products containing sugar and GMOs? Why does the FDA back medicine with terrifying side effects while insisting on adding devaluing warning labels to natural products with no known side effects besides actually healing consumers? Is Watergate possibly one example of corruption in our own government? This isn't conspiracy theorems; we're challenging you to critical thinking.

Information plus application equals transformation. We're giving you the information, it's your job to apply it. Should you decide to take that step you can expect a transformation in your health.

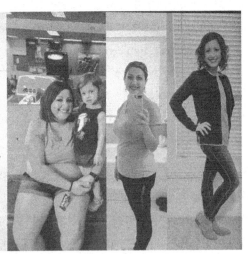

JENNIFER

- **LOST 95 pounds!**
- Increased **Energy!**
- Neck Pain EXTREMELY **decreased!**
- **Headaches** significantly reduced

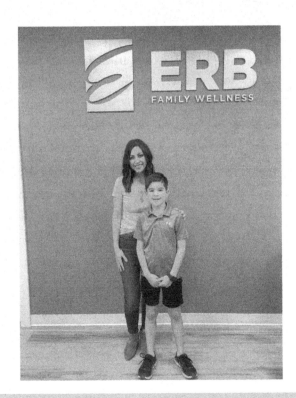

My mom-in-law and her friend suggested we go see the Erbs. My son was having some behavioral issues and ticks. He also gets migraines.

Initially I wasn't thinking about my own health. We were getting my son adjusted and the Erbs were giving me a lot of things we could try at home to help him overcome. Nutrition was a big part of our transformation. The way I cook has completely changed. I also became a sugar Nazi. I eliminated it form my family's diet realizing that the result doesn't outweigh the reward. My son's ticks are now mostly nonexistent, and his migraines are better too.

As a result of getting my son the help he needs, I began to care for myself too. I have been in multiple car accidents and had herniated disks. I almost always had migraine headaches and I was constantly tired. I was set to have disk fusion surgery, but I put it off. That's another reason my mother-in-law suggested we go see the Erbs.

My diet changed along with my son's, and I too started getting my spine adjusted. I lost almost 100 pounds! I began to get my energy back! My migraines began to decrease as well. It's been about two years since we started, but in February 2020 I experienced a setback. I was hit on my side of the car by a high schooler while my kids were with me. It restarted my whole road to recovery again, except this time it's been so much better having Erb Family Wellness from the start. As of the last 6-8 months the pain and subluxation has dramatically improved. The Erbs have been a light, especially in these dark times. – Jennifer Keller

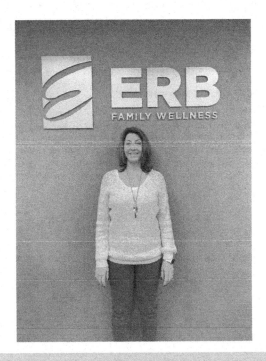

When I first started going to Erb Family Wellness I was sleeping less than four hours a night. For the past year, before I began my treatment with them, my whole body ached, and I was sore all the time. I was irritable and moody. My colon wasn't functioning at all. I came with some major issues in my neck and mid to lower back. I felt full and bloated all the time. No matter what I did I could not lose weight whether not eating, diet or exercise. Nothing worked.

The night after my very first spinal adjustment I slept like a baby all night long! That had not happened in years. Getting a good night's sleep has been the biggest impact for me but coupling chiropractic care with the metabolic test has been life changing.

Dr. Kimberly told me to give her six months for my customized program based on my metabolic test and my X-rays to get to a healthier place. I'm about three months into my treatment and have been consistent to get adjusted, take my supplements, change my diet including eating more.

I'm already feeling much better and I'm getting better each day. The inflammation is diminishing, and my bowels are much more consistent. I've also started losing weight! My husband says, "You aren't moody anymore." It's true, since I have been feeling better and more energetic, my passion to help others has returned.

I could not be more thrilled. I'm looking forward to my next appointment and taking my health to the next level. – Lori Little

# CHAPTER 3
# BITTERSWEET
# SEDUCTION

"Do you like honey? Don't eat too much, or it will make you sick!"

Proverbs 25:16 NLT

"For the lips of an immoral woman drip honey, And her mouth *is* smoother than oil." Proverbs 5:3 NLT warns of the seductive words spoken not only by an "immoral woman," but by other unethical people as well. Every day, everywhere we turn, we are being enticed to give into our lust for something sweet. We and our children are being seduced by the marketing of a deadly substance as addictive as opioids.

The nearly $100 billion sugar industry is banking on our naive response to its message while the USDA continues to recommend its high-carb, low-fat diet. Meanwhile, obesity and diabetes are on the rise.

## Dodging Disease

Consuming sugar is like crossing a freeway during rush hour. Vehicles big and small are coming at you. You may make it to the other side, but you're more likely to be hit by something. Whether it's liver disease, heart disease, cancer, hormone imbalances, inflammation, a weakened immune system, or diabetes, consuming sugar puts you at risk for developing one or more of these diseases.

One study found that those who ate more than 25% of their daily calories from sugar were two times more likely to die from heart disease compared to those who only had 10% or fewer calories from sugar.

Even if you wouldn't describe yourself as having a sweet tooth, sugar is hidden in 74% of packaged foods—and simple carbs like white flour, white rice and potatoes also turn into glucose or sugar making diabetes an accident waiting to happen.

Your body uses insulin to move sugar into the cells for energy rather than leaving it in the bloodstream. The constant traffic of sugar causes the insulin receptors on the cells to burn out resulting in insulin resistance. When the body's ability to produce or respond to the hormone insulin is impaired, resulting in abnormal metabolism of carbohydrates and elevated levels of glucose in the blood and urine, it results in a diabetes diagnosis.

Every day 4,460 Americans are diagnosed with diabetes. With the continued syrupy marketing of sugar, this disease is a growing issue in our country. It has risen from 108 million diagnosed in 1980 to 422 million in 2014. Equally alarming, about one in four adults with diabetes don't even know they have it! That's not even counting the 86 million Americans who have *pre*diabetes.

Diabetes and prediabetes cost America $322 million per year. Those diagnosed with diabetes pay 2.3 times more for healthcare costs than those without the disease. That's not so sweet.

Besides the guilty pleasure of eating sugar, other risk factors for being hit with a diabetes diagnosis are:

- Family history of diabetes
- Risk increases over age 45
- Insulin resistant syndrome (tired after eating)
- Obesity
- Hispanics, Blacks, Native Americans and Asians have a greater risk

- Inactivity or lack of exercise
- Abnormal cholesterol levels
- History of gestational diabetes

- High blood pressure

The American Diabetes Association offers very little hope, stating that "diabetes is a progressive disease requiring more medication over time." It doesn't sound like the insulin therapy doctrine provides any hope for salvation from this disease. Insulin therapy doesn't treat the cause nor cure diabetes, nor does it prevent the disease from progressing; it actually **increases** risk of cancer and cardiovascular events! "The overall results of this meta-analysis do not show a benefit of intensive glucose lowering treatment on all-cause mortality or cardiovascular death. A 19% increase in all-cause mortality and a 43% increase in cardiovascular mortality cannot be excluded" (British Medical Journal). Simply stated, insulin therapy by itself causes more death, not less.

The Chemical Religion wanted to cash in on the diabetes opportunity, so they concocted a pill. *Avandia* was on the market in 1999, but in 2007 the New England Journal of Medicine reported that there was a 43% increased risk of heart attack and 64% higher risk of cardiovascular death on the prescribed drug. More than 80,000 of the drug's victims suffered strokes, heart failure and other complications. I wonder if M.D.s were unaware of these horrendous results as they continued to prescribe the dangerous medication for the next 10 years it took to restrict its use?

As with all prescription drugs, the other meds used in insulin therapy (such as Metformin, Sulfonylureas, Meglitinides, Thiazolidinediones, DPP-4 Inhibitors, GLP-1 receptor agonists, SGLT1 inhibitors) all come with dangerous side-effects. Drugs aren't the cure, and neither are the "diabetic supplies" being pushed in grocery stores with long lists of unpronounceable and toxic ingredients. Big Business can afford expensive marketing meant to seduce the naïve.

Diabetes isn't the only danger that accompanies too much sugar in your bloodstream. High blood sugar comes with further health risks including kidney, eye and heart disease. Insulin resistance is the biggest risk factor for heart disease and is associated with accelerated aging. If those trucks don't hit you, nerve damage or stroke might.

### Repelling the Seduction

Only recently is the truth coming out with the popularity of diets like Keto, Paleo and Hunter-Gatherer. It's proven that good fats protect against cognitive impairment and reduce the risk of cardiovascular and neurodegenerative diseases. People are finally able to lose weight, think more clearly, overcome or better manage diabetes, and are experiencing overall greater health.

It is not surprising that medical professionals, the USDA and the FDA are not the ones preaching this gospel. It's regular people, who haven't found the answers they were looking for in medicine, who are going against the flow, bucking the USDA's food pyramid concept and inspiring others to a healthier way of eating. In fact, their voice has grown so strong that it's forcing the food industry to change. Or at least, it's forcing them to change the way the industry markets their products. So be warned: they've learned how to sound healthy with labels boasting *organic, free range, gluten free, less sugar, half the calories, all natural* ... you get the idea. While still appealing to America's sweet tooth, artificial sweeteners have replaced the addictive substance that has captivated so many by smooth-talking marketing.

## Is Artificial Sweet Safer?

In the late 90's the FDA's own toxicologist, Dr. Adrian Gross, told Congress that without a shadow of a doubt aspartame can cause brain tumors and brain cancer. Top doctors and researchers confirmed that aspartame causes headaches, memory loss, seizures, vision loss, comas and cancer. It worsens or mimics the symptoms of such diseases and conditions as fibromyalgia, MS, lupus, ADD, diabetes, Alzheimer's, chronic fatigue and depression. Aspartame also liberates free methyl alcohol resulting in chronic methanol poisoning, affecting the dopamine system of the brain and causing *addiction*. Methanol, or wood alcohol, constitutes one third of the aspartame molecule and is classified as a severe metabolic *poison* and *narcotic*.

Aspartame, not surprisingly was once owned by Monsanto, changed its name to AminoSweet as awareness of its harmful effects became more known. In their quest to be thin many consumers continue to partake of diet foods and beverages containing this deadly substance, while it's actually making them fat! Research has shown that drinking diet sodas increase risk of metabolic syndrome, which may double the risk of obesity. It also stimulates an appetite, which is obviously not a dieter's dream.

## What to Buy?

Simply stated, buy things that don't come with labels, but when you must, look for labels that say, "Non-GMO" and "Certified Organic". Also, don't bother trying to sound out ingredients with long, complicated names. If it's difficult to pronounce it's probably not a natural ingredient. Just put the item back on the shelf. Don't be fooled by the marketing meant to distract you from reading the ingredients. Maybe these catchy phrases will come to mind as you stroll the isles:

- Fresh is best.

- Packaged is poor.

- Can't read it, don't eat it.

- Artificial and unnatural are inedible.

- Fat is fine.

## What Do I Eat?

Changing your diet isn't as hard as changing your *mind* about your diet. Of course, there are some things you need to eliminate, but think of it as an adventure or an exploration! There are so many delicious foods and recipes you've yet to experience. We'll help you find them in chapter 13.

You'll need to let go of grains, sugars and most fruit. Sadly, even healthy grains rapidly turn to sugar. You'll also need to moderate your intake of protein. While we advocate for keto diets, sometimes people can get carried away and consume too much protein. Not everyone realizes that excessive protein can also turn into sugar called gluconeogenesis. Men should have 25-35 grams per meal. Women need approximately 25 grams of protein per meal. Also: remove bad fats. (See Appendix for which fats to avoid)

After you've detoxed your frig and cabinets, fill them back up with these:

- Stevia or erythritol instead of sugar or artificial sweeteners

- Low glycemic fruits like berries, grapefruit and granny smith apples

- Grass-fed, free-range, antibiotic-free beef, bison, chicken, eggs

- rBGH free milk

- Non-farm raised fish

- Quality whey protein from 100% naturally raised cows

- No hormones or pesticides

- Good fats such as olive oil, coconut oil & products, avocados, nuts such as walnuts and almonds and Omega-3 fatty acids

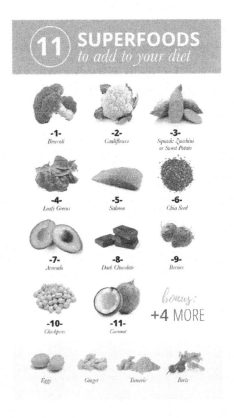

Dr. Roy Taylor told *Diabetologia* that Type 2 diabetes can be reversed within one-to-eight weeks through diet changes. He said, "The bottom line: A dramatic diet change in diabetics reversed most features of diabetes within one week and all features by eight weeks." Dr. Taylor continued, "That's right, diabetes was reversed in one week. That's more powerful than any drug known to modern science."

Seductive marketing deceives us into sickness. Read the list of ingredients or you'll be consuming products that lead you back to the pharmacy. Don't be fooled by the Chemical Religion, there's no quick fix for your body's scary response to the toxic foods you bought into. Symptoms are your body's way of getting your attention. Your body is trying to tell you it's hungry for real food and a healthier lifestyle.

## Exercise Bursting with Benefits

The best way to predict the future is to create it. Who will you be in five to ten years? Will you be on multiple medications, having regular hospital visits and facing a scary prognosis? Will you still be ensnared by the smooth lips of marketing appeals dripping of sweet lies? Or will you do what it takes to be a healthier, happier, stronger you? Disenchanting from the seduction starts with getting your power back, and there's no better way to become powerful than to start exercising!

Never underestimate the power of exercise to avoid or overcome diseases, including diabetes. Treat it like it's your prescription for health. Take the "exercise pill" as religiously as you might have if it had been one given to you by your M.D. The side effects are the results you've been praying for!

The American Heart Association Meeting Report praised short bursts of high-intensity exercise for its impact on Type 2 diabetes. In fact, exercise proved to be far superior to the popular diabetes drug Metformin by three-to-one in a relatively large study of over 3000 obese individuals over 25 years of age with impaired glucose tolerance.

Short-term sprint intervals increase insulin sensitivity, so your body doesn't have to produce as much. Also (without getting too technical) the mitochondria are the energy engines within every cell. Exercise makes them work better and increases the number. The effects of these workouts on insulin and the mitochondria increase energy and focus naturally without the use of the Chemical Religion's potions.

Short bursts of high-intensity exercise provide greater results than sustaining 30 minutes of lower-intensity exercise. Burst exercise gives Type 2 diabetes patients more than a two-fold greater improvement in HbA1c levels, a measure of blood sugar levels. It also improves cholesterol and body mass index.

Changing your diet and exercising offers more hope for avoiding diabetes or recovering from it than popping a bunch of pills. In fact, insulin resistance therapy only offers higher and higher dosages.

Mark Hyman, M.D., exhorts, "This is a disease that is nearly 100 percent preventable and reversible. But it won't be solved in the doctor's office, clinic or hospital. It has to be fixed where it begins: in our homes, communities and our society and in our government policies and industry practices. This is a social disease, and we need a social cure."

When it's produced naturally food is meant to fuel and heal the body. At least at some point it should have been alive and growing rather than formulated in a lab. Diabetes and other diseases don't have to be a life sentence. Changing the way you move and the way you eat can change your future.

Let's get physical and free from the seduction! Now that's sexy!

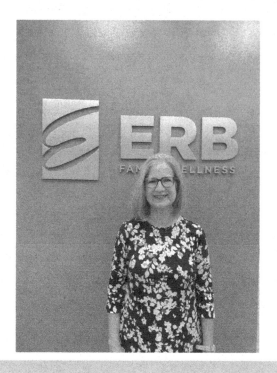

I started with the Erbs around June of 2013 or so. I have my daughter to thank for inviting me to a community dinner where Dr. Erb was sharing. I learned very quickly that my idea of health and nutrition was backwards. For example, the over-the-counter meds I thought were safe were not. Spending money on quality food has become important to me since I've been coming to Erb Family Wellness.

First of all, in getting acquainted with the five health values they teach, spinal adjustments and the way I eat made the biggest impact for me. To stay on course when I travel, I needed to find chiropractors I could go to while away. I also took my traction equipment with me so that I could continue my home spinal exercises. I was once questioned about the suspicious looking gadgets by TSA on my way to Israel.

I've experienced significant injuries and have been thankful to be a patient of Dr. Erb. I have had three falls since being under their care.

I have injured my elbow, tailbone and sternum. Consistent adjustments have made the difference in my recovery.

I attribute my ability to have overcome shingles, hives and vertigo so quickly to the open-door policy at Erb Family Wellness. It seems so counter intuitive to "come on in" when I am sick, but the Erbs encourage sick patients to come in more when they are fighting something off. I believe adjustments and vitamin D are really what got me back on my feet more quickly. They have made a huge difference!

It's really important to me to be able to take care of my grandchildren; to swing them around and put them in a cart. A number of people say they see me as healthier and stronger than others that are my age. I might fall off the food or adjustment wagon, but I can get right back on. Every day is a new day.

Erb Family Wellness certainly has been a place of "hope and healing" for me. – Lianne Wynne

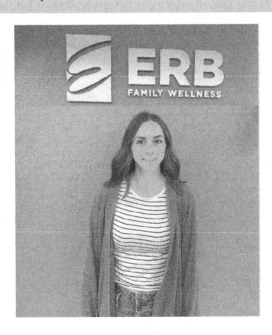

I've been going to Erb Family Wellness for about a year. I had been vegan for 7 years when I started going for chiropractic care. I began feeling fatigued, having brain fog, anxiety and not well overall. My diet had been vegan for so long that I would not have expected it to be my problem even as I watched the Erbs' videos on proper nutrition.

All of a sudden it just hit me, and it was a huge crash. My symptoms increased, so I did metabolic testing and found that my body type especially needs protein. It indicated that I was also deficient in many vitamins. My vegan diet consisted of lots of fruit and carbs, so it was really high in sugar.

I did everything Dr. Kimberly told me to do including changing my diet and taking supplements to give my body the nourishment it had been missing. I am no longer fatigued. I can think clearly, and the anxiety is gone. Feeling better has renewed my desire to reach out to help others. Now that my body is getting what it needs, I am also gaining muscle when I work out which is something I couldn't do before. – Lindsey Edmonds

# CHAPTER 4
# TIME FOR A CHANGE
# OF HEART

"For as he thinks in his heart, so *is* he. 'Eat and drink!' he says to you, but his heart is not with you." Proverbs 23:7 NKJV

"Your heart is dying in your chest." I can still remember the cardiologist's words like it was yesterday. The hopelessness I faced led me to the destiny I'm fulfilling.

As far as I knew, I wasn't at risk. I ate well and stayed active. In fact, I was kind of an athletic superstar doing tricks on skis and skateboards. But like most of us who haven't experienced a health scare, I didn't really understand the risk factors for heart disease. But I've learned there's a lot of misinformation about it coming from the medical industry, so let me be clear. Here are the actual risk factors leading to heart disease.

- Smoking/vaping
- Diabetes

- Overweight

- Poor diet and sugar

- Physical inactivity

- Excessive alcohol use

- High blood pressure

- Inflammation

- Stress

- Low cholesterol (What? I'll explain later how low cholesterol is dangerous.)

- Statins (Yes, pills that are supposed to prevent heart disease can cause it.)

- NSAID's (Over-the-counter pain meds increase risk by more than 50%)

- **Subluxation** (This is an important one that the M.D.s aren't talking about)

The medical industry talks a lot about genetics playing a big role in heart disease, but the truth is they're only a small factor. Bruce Lipton says, "Genes load the gun; lifestyle pulls the trigger." I knew I came from good genes and my lifestyle was exemplary, but the thing I didn't know about heart health was the thing that eventually saved me.

## How Does My Spine Impact My Heart and Health?

Years before my symptoms began, I walked away pain-free from a car accident. I thought I was fine, but the loss of the proper curve in my neck was cutting off the nerve, blood and oxygen supply to my heart. When I met for that long dinner with the chiropractor who educated Kimberly and me, ultimately saving my life, he explained subluxation to me. It didn't matter how fit I was or how healthy I ate, if the bones in my spine were pinching off the nerve supply to my organs, I was going to get sick eventually.

Subluxation occurs when the spine suffers abnormalities that cause interference with the nervous system. After reviewing my x-rays, my chiropractor, who happened to be my wife, discovered that my spine had been damaged from the auto accident. She explained that my vertebrae protects my spinal column which is connected to every part of my body including my heart. My beautiful D.C. used my x-rays and a chart to show me the location of my subluxation and which organs were affected. My heart was dying because it had been cut off from the life-giving supply pinched between my vertebrates. Just like a plant withers and dies without water, our organs cannot survive cut off from their sustaining source.

After only a few adjustments my symptoms were gone but I continued treatment until my spine was completely corrected. Even years later, I continue to get regular adjustments to maintain my excellent health.

My wife and I have discovered layer upon layer deceptions that are making people sick. Greed has made true health the Chemical Religion's best kept secret.

### Has Heart Disease Become a Money-Making Opportunity?

The proverb warns about the ones encouraging us to "eat and drink though their heart isn't with us." They don't care about us in the same way that the food industry is heartlessly marketing toxic foods to us while being fully aware of the harmful ingredients. Unsuspectingly we serve everyday products like ketchup, fruit juice, lunch meats and breads to our kids all containing sugar that cause a host of chronic diseases, including heart disease. If we want to change our heart health, we have to first change our mind about what we put our faith in.

Heart Disease is another money-making killer in the U.S. It accounts for:

- 1 out of 3 deaths

- 1 death every 38 seconds

- $1.1 trillion by 2035

This is no longer just a concern for the more mature adults. The New England Journal of Medicine reported that when 200 youth were autopsied after being involved in fatal accidents, 10% of the kids already had fibrous plaquing of their coronary arteries. In the autopsied group between the ages of 16 to 20, 35% had plaquing in the arteries. By the mid 20's age group, over 70% had plaquing of the arteries. Kids love sugar, but just like other dangerous drugs from which we try to protect our children, sugar is a deadly addiction.

*Journal Watch* in 2008 that the American Academy of Pediatrics (AAP) had issued new guidelines for lipid screening and cholesterol management in children after growing concerns. One recommendation has eyebrows raising among physicians and consumer health advocates who understand the risks associated with giving children drugs designed for adults.

Cholesterol drugs are already on our radar for being intrusive to the body's natural self-healing process, but subjecting *children* as young as *eight* years old is a huge red flag for most in the healthcare profession. That is, of course, with the exception of the pharmaceutical companies. They will greatly benefit financially if they can convince M.D.s to prescribe their products to trusting families rather than teach parents how to combat the potential for heart disease with diet and exercise.

Besides Big Pharma's plan to increase statin sales through prescriptions to children, they've also tweaked some numbers in their favor. The old definition of high cholesterol was 240 but that wasn't making enough money, so the pharmaceutical companies pushed to lower what is considered high cholesterol to 200. The change made an 86% increase from nearly 48.5

million statins prescribed to over 92 million prescribed. How much more money do you think they made?

A conservative cost estimate for cholesterol-reducing medications is $150 for a month's supply, paid out-of-pocket and through insurance. Multiply that by the difference 43,647,000 and the industry just increased their sales more than $6.5 billion. While Big Pharma is increasing their bottom line, we're taking their pills and creating more health issues for ourselves. Imagine how much more money they could make if they could convince doctors to prescribe to kids?

There are a lot of people walking around on meds they don't need. For instance, many women have been unnecessarily put on cholesterol meds because they were tested at the wrong end of their menstrual cycle. Women's cholesterol spikes just after they start their period, and it dips just before they start. So, if a woman happens to go in for her routine visit while her cholesterol is on the higher side, how likely is it that her non OBGYN doctor will ask her where she is in her cycle? I've never heard of it happening. It's much more likely a prescription will be given along with a little dose of fear.

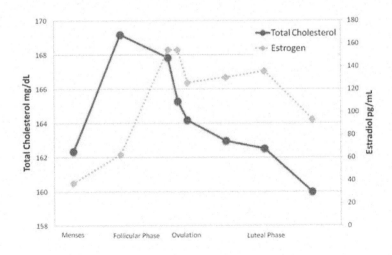

There are a lot of factors that can change the numbers. Before you agree to start popping these pills ask yourself a few questions. Have you suffered a loss? Have you been under stress or had a car accident? Have you been getting enough sleep or been food binging? All of these temporary circumstances can change your numbers, but once managed your cholesterol will come back into balance on its own. Heightened cholesterol serves a purpose. It's not your body misfunctioning.

Contrary to what you've been taught by the medical doctrine, cholesterol is necessary to the health and function of your body.

### What is it and Why Do I Need it?

Cholesterol is a soft waxy substance mostly produced by our liver. It's carried through our bloodstream as either HDL or LDL. Without it our body cannot make hormones or vitamin D which might be why we are seeing so many low testosterone and fem centers opening up. Statins force cholesterol down, decreasing their body's ability to produce necessary building blocks to their health.

Men taking the drug can't understand why they're struggling with erectile dysfunction and are losing muscle. Even though doctors prescribe statins knowing the side effects of the drug, when their patients come back explaining their frustrations in the bedroom and with their softer body, patients are told that it's their age and to consider hormone pellets (thus the popularity of Low-T centers).

Women taking statins suffer similarly with decreased energy, sex drive and loss of figure. They're diagnosed premenopausal and more drugs are recommended such as hormone replacement therapy, which of course come with another set of undesirable side effects.

Cholesterol meds also block the body's ability to produce CoQ10, an important antioxidant needed to transfer energy from food to our cells.

It helps to reduce inflammation and protects us from cancer and aging. It's also the primary building block for the cells in our brain and nervous system. Blocking it often causes what is called by the M.D.s who prescribe the meds, "Statin Induced Dementia." In fact, there's even a diagnosis code (ICD-10 T46.6X5A) assigned to the condition.

Also, CoQ10 levels have been found to be low in people with heart disease, which would seem to indicate another reason why statins increase risk for developing the disease. That's a pretty hard pill to swallow!

Another helpful function compromised by statins is the extra cholesterol produced that wraps around an injury to protect it as it heals. Cholesterol has been misunderstood for too long as something we must battle within our own body while the drugs prescribed to combat it are destroying our health pill by pill.

Statins are anything but harmless. They work by inhibiting a vital enzyme that manufactures cholesterol in the liver (HMG-C0A). Although the brain represents only 2% of our total body weight it contains 25% of the body's cholesterol! The brain and nerve tissue will begin to deteriorate when cholesterol is lowered with statins. They also cause depression by blocking serotonin uptake sites which decrease serotonin. Furthermore, they cause liver damage, neuropathy (numbness and tingling in extremities), severe joint pain, ligament rupture, atrophy and heart failure.

High cholesterol can become a concern but avoiding fats and taking drugs isn't the answer. Dr. William P. Castelli, who analyzed data from a long-term Framingham study in 1992, found that the more saturated fat people ate, the *lower* their serum cholesterol was. That doesn't mean we can go crazy eating food from drive-throughs. Consuming healthy fats like coconut and fish oils help regulate cholesterol naturally rather than blocking it all together creating other health risks.

Another surprising fact about cholesterol is that low cholesterol can be more dangerous than high. The European Heart Journal examined 11,500 patients and found those with cholesterol below 160 were more than twice as likely to die than those with high cholesterol! The National Cancer Institute backed a study of 12,488 men and women and found that men with the lowest cholesterol levels were most likely to get cancer.

The bottom line is that pills are not the answer. Studies have shown that, in total mortality, statins make no difference in those who are at-risk for heart disease compared to those taking placebo pills. Researchers followed 114 patients with heart problems who began taking cholesterol lowering drugs and found that every point of decrease of the serum cholesterol, there was a 36% increase in risk of death from heart attacks.

### Keeping a Happy Heart

Don't let stress put you at risk for heart disease. Everyone has stress, but if stress is left unmanaged and prolonged it can be a risk factor. Studies have linked stress to heart disease, obesity, asthma, diabetes, depression, gastro-intestinal issues and accelerated aging.

High blood pressure causes medical patients much alarm, but the definitions for hypertension have also been adjusted, giving it a 35% increase in new high blood pressure diagnoses—and an increase in Big Pharma's bottom line. The numbers can be scary unless you understand how blood pressure works and that there isn't a one-size-fits-all range.

"Normal" blood pressure is said to be 120 over 80, but the bigger the body, the higher the blood pressure needs to be to pump the blood from the feet all the way back up to the brain. A tiny woman has much less distance to travel than that of a large man. You may not realize that our body will adjust to our size; so, for each pound of fat gained, our body will create a new network of seven miles of blood vessels. To put that in perspective, if you gain ten fatty pounds you will now have 70 extra miles of blood vessels.

It's easy to see why obesity and heart disease go together. If you want to decrease your blood pressure, taking meds that have been found to actually increase the risk of stroke offer fewer desirable results than simply changing your diet and exercising. Get the weight off and decrease your risk of heart disease.

George Howard, Doctor of Public Health, and a professor in the Department of Biostatistics in the UAB School of Public Health, led a team of researchers from the University of Alabama at Birmingham. They published in the journal *Stroke* that "the risk of stroke went up 33 percent with each blood pressure medicine required to treat blood pressure to goal. Compared to people with systolic blood pressure below 120 mmHg without treatment, hypertensive individuals on three or more blood pressure medications had a stroke risk of 2.5 times higher."

The study indicates that there is no benefit in adding additional blood pressure medications. **The more meds the greater the risk.**

"The way to curb the problem," Howard says, "is to prevent hypertension in the first place." My wife and I teach our patients five practices that prevent and heal diseases. We call them the Gospels of Good Health (We'll explain these keys in greater detail in Chapter 13.)

- Hope Filled Mind
- Tap Into God's Power Source
- Get Back to the Garden
- Breath In Energy
- Repent of Toxins

By God's design, even when arteries become blocked our body is so smart that it will actually make a new pathway. So, if heart disease is a concern, you can risk prescription drugs, bypass surgery and have a stint put in. Or you can do what I did and get your spine corrected, get your lifestyle in check with diet, exercise, stress management and plenty of rest. Your body will do the rest. When I returned to the cardiologist, he was bewildered by the fact it looked like I had a brand-new heart.

Don't be discouraged if you're already on meds. We're here to offer you hope. You can get your health back. As you make some changes you can work with your M.D. to decrease your dosages or, if necessary, find another doctor who is willing to work with you. There's nothing to feel ashamed of for having been misled by society's methods and marketing. The fact that you're reading this book indicates that you're seeking the truth. You're seeking a change.

Sometimes our greatest tragedies can actually propel us to *become* who we were created to be. In times of crisis, we search for answers, and when we find them, we become passionate to share the hope we've found with others. Kimberly and I are dedicated to empowering people to get healthy and to find freedom from the Chemical Religion.

"It is for freedom that Christ has set us free. Stand firm, then, and do not
let yourselves be burdened again by a yoke of slavery."
Galatians 5:1 NIV

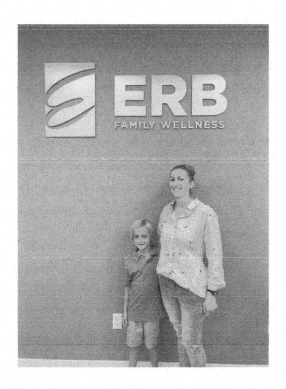

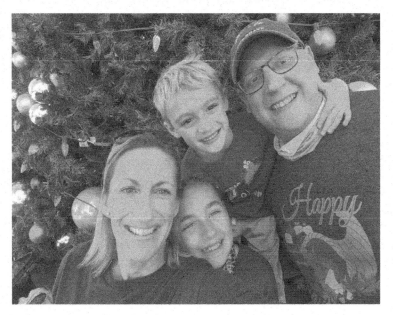

When I was pregnant with my daughter, I was told that I had cardiomyopathy (heart failure). I was so swollen! My lips were swollen. My ankles were as big as my thighs! To make matters worse, I had preeclampsia. The pregnancy and delivery were very difficult. I pushed for 24 hours.

I was told that I would die if I ever tried to have another baby. We saw an OB specialist who went so far as to write a letter that he would not consent for us to get pregnant again. We sought help from a cardiologist who put me on medications that made me extremely tired and ill. Scarlett was three months old, and I would fall asleep playing with her. I eventually just stopped taking the drugs.

Scarlett got pneumonia when she was four years old. The medical doctors said she would never be active. They said she would always have breathing issues. That was just before we started going to the Erbs'.

My husband and I went to a dinner where Dr. David shared his story of heart sickness and that's what made us decide to seek his care. The spinal adjustments corrected my posture and made a huge difference along with changing my eating habits. I began eating the way they teach to cleanse my body from all the toxic meds, and I continued to be consistent with my usual workouts.

We waited 6 months to a year for my body to recover while under Dr. David's care before planning our next baby. It was the easiest pregnancy compared to our first experience. I was adjusted all though my pregnancy. I didn't have heart issues or preeclampsia and I could not believe how quickly the delivery went.

Scarlett also began getting adjustments. Today she is a very healthy and active child who plays sports. She doesn't suffer from asthma or other breathing problems.

We have a healthy, miracle son thanks to Erb Family Wellness! – Amy DiPasquale

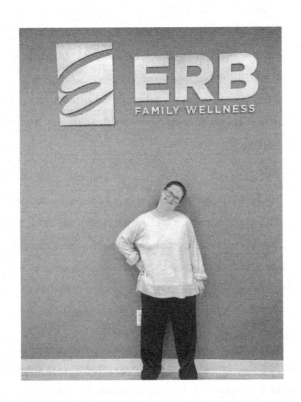

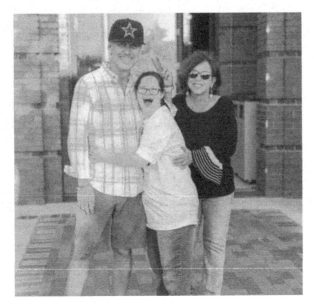

We started going to Erb Family Wellness 2 ½ years ago. A lady joined our Bible study group the night we were praying for our daughter who has down syndrome. Molly struggled to walk on her own. Two surgeons were highly recommending she have surgery. Our new friend said, "I really want you to see my doctor. I think he can help you." When I realized her doctor was a chiropractor I thought, "Oh my gosh, I have done chiropractors before."

Turns out the Erbs aren't like any other chiropractor we've been to before. After the first two weeks of getting adjusted, we took Molly to a local concert. She got up and started dancing for two hours! We had taken Molly to an Elvis impersonator concert just the December before. She loves Elvis's music, but she sat and cried in her chair from the pain and discomfort. The difference Dr. David made was a miracle. We canceled the surgery after we saw her dancing. My husband and I said to each other, "We aren't going to need to do this."

We were all in on this Erb Family Wellness care in less than two months. We went to their makeover classes about nutrition and spinal care. That's when a light bulb went off for us. Between the two of us, we had been on meds for arthritis, blood pressure and acid reflux. From that day on we started eating from their most beneficial diet plan and within a month we were both losing weight. We later added exercise to our routine—I lost 30 pounds and my husband lost 64 within the first six months and have managed to keep it off during the last two and a half years! Even Molly has continued to lose weight.

We were also able to get off our medications with the help of the Erbs and under the supervision of our medical doctors. Molly was on 13 pills. She had been taking a thyroid pill for 20 years! We reduced it until the MD agreed we could take her. She has been able to maintain her levels within normal ranges.

The year before we came to Erb Family Wellness, the doctor was afraid Molly was going to have to have heart surgery. She had already had open heart surgery at 4 years old and again at 18. Every year we go to the cardiologist to have her checked. Her primary doctor and the cardiologist said, "I don't know what you are doing but her heart function is so much better than it was the year before."

Our family continues to stick to the healthy diet plan, and we are still going for our adjustments because we realize how important it all is. We're still learning and going to the Erbs' classes. This is just a part of our lifestyle now. Molly knows that Dr. David healed her back. She calls him her superman. - Sherrie Hawk

# CHAPTER 5
# DEFUNDING CANCER:
# UNCOVERING THE
# HIDDEN CURE

"For the love of money is a root of all *kinds of* evil, for which some have strayed from the faith in their greediness and pierced themselves through with many sorrows."

1 Timothy 6:10 NKJ

When we were growing up cancer was barely ever mentioned. HIV was the disease getting all the attention and funding. But as the microwave generation evolved, turning to convenience foods filled with sugar and additives, eventually cancer made a name for itself as a deadly disease that could strike at any moment. No one knew what caused it, how to protect themselves from it or who its next victim would be.

## Where Does All That Money Go?

The National Cancer Institute defines cancer: "A term for diseases in which abnormal cells divide without control and can invade nearby tissues. Cancer cells can also spread to other parts of the body through the blood and lymph systems." It's the body's natural immune response when it is unsuccessful in combatting the rapid production of damaged or disease-causing cells.

The cancer industry isn't hurting financially. In 1995 studies estimated cancer cost the United States over $96 billion. At least 260 nonprofits are raising money for research. The National Cancer Institute alone has spent $90 billion on research since the war on cancer was declared. In spite of all the money spent on its exploration, medical science still seems to know very little.

Marketing meant to fuel our fear of cancer has made the pharmaceutical companies a lot of money while the business of food seems to be facilitating a continued need for answers. Most of us know someone who has suffered and died from this mysterious disease, leaving us easily manipulated into donating to the bottomless pit in hopes that it will be the dollar that finally brings hope.

To get to the heart of a matter, follow the money. Breast Cancer Awareness was a clever marketing plan created by the pharmaceutical company AstraZeneca. Komen's Race to the Cure isn't much better. About 95% of the donation money goes to provide free mammograms to African American women and low-income women, rather than to research. Investing in women who might not be able to afford testing seems admirable, but we'll explain later how the motives are still from a heart of greed.

Whether you donate your money to their cause or to any of the countless others, you're giving money to one of the most bloated industries in the world. Face it: we have been racing for the cure since 1983 but as long as the founders keep raking in the dough there's still no finish line in sight.

Nevertheless, that doesn't mean we're helpless in the face of cancer statistics. Our friend, Dr. Charlie Majors, who spent his life researching and fighting cancer says, "the cause is the cure." If we want to overcome cancer, we need to discover the cause.

## What Grows Cancer?

Cancer *craves* sugar! We all have a few sick cells, but until they begin to reproduce and accumulate, they're not called cancer. Making sugar a part of your daily diet is like nourishing weeds in your garden that will grow to choke out what you've planted. Cancer cells feed off sugar and use the fermentation process for energy to rapidly multiply. Excessive consumption causes insulin resistance, leading to inflammation and all kinds of diseases.

Even refined carbs like white flour, white rice and potatoes are linked to increased cancer risk because of their high glycemic index. They basically turn into sugar when you eat them. These carbs are rapidly digested and cause quick blood sugar spikes. Foods with a high glycemic index have been linked to an 88% higher risk of developing prostate cancer and an increased risk of developing other cancers.

Dr. Lewis Cantley, a Harvard Researcher, studies sugar and cancer. His research has proven that many cancer cells have insulin receptors on their surface that 'hi-jack' sugar (glucose) and use that sugar to grow the tumor. Even PET scans prove cancer's need for it. To detect where cancer is, a doctor will inject radioactive sugar into patients where it will be pulled into the cancer like a magnet revealing its location. Almost immediately, sugar decreases the function of our immune system, which is detrimental when trying to kick cancer.

It just seems logical that the first step to fighting cancer is to starve it by cutting out sugar, but how often is that a part of the conversation in a medical facility?

## What Can We Do to Protect Ourselves?

The current dogma that cancer is a genetic disease isn't quite true. Like we said before, "genes load the gun, lifestyle pulls the trigger." Cleaning up your lifestyle is like engaging the safety on the gun. It won't fire if the safety is on. Exercise, eliminating sugar, managing stress and getting spinal adjustments are our best protection from becoming cancer's next statistic. Keeping our lifestyle, diet and environment in check empowers us to engage our safety button. Lower your risks with these tips:

- **Lifestyle**: stress, obesity, lack of sleep, lack of sunlight, lack of physical activity.

- **Diet:** too much sugar, too many refined carbohydrates, vegetable oils and trans fats, lack of anti-cancer foods and lack of probiotics and prebiotics.

- **Environment:** tobacco and alcohol, endocrine disruptors, GMOs, rBGH and the use of toxic sunscreen.

Exercise is like a breath of fresh air to our cells! Unlike cancer cells that are non-aerobic, meaning they function without oxygen, healthy cells function aerobically. They love oxygen! Exercise gets our heart rate up causing us to take in more of this life-giving air.

Exercise has been shown to decrease cancer risk by reducing inflammation, reducing stress, regulating hormones and improving the immune system. Low, moderate and intense exercise boosts our number of disease-fighting-immunity cells improving our immune system as long as we aren't overstressing our body. Even simply walking for thirty minutes a day decreases breast cancer risk by 60%!

Otto Warburg is considered one of the 20th century's leading biochemists. He was the sole recipient of the Nobel Prize in Physiology and Medicine in

1931. In total, he was nominated for the award 47 times over the course of his career. Published in the article *The Root Cause of Cancer* he said, "The root cause of cancer is oxygen deficiency, which creates an acidic state in the human body." He taught that cancer cannot survive in the presence of high levels of oxygen, as found in an alkaline state. In frustration, when his findings were ignored or rejected, Warburg often quoted Max Planck, "Science advances one funeral at a time."

How do we fight cancer? Proper nutrition and a diet such as one that is ketogenic alleviates our risk for certain cancers and diseases. According to Dr. Thomas Seyfried, author of *Cancer as a Metabolic Disease*, our body is always producing ketones, but they replace glucose as our body's primary energy source in ketosis, therefore starving cancerous cells. Adding low-glycemic foods to your diet such as fruits and vegetables have been associated with a 67% lower risk of developing breast cancer, especially cruciferous vegetables like broccoli and cauliflower that are actually known cancer-fighting foods. Dr. Seyfried said in an interview with Dr. Kara Fitzgerald, "It [cancer] will grow as fast as it can as long as fuels are available. Targeting the fuels that these cells use to grow seems like a very logical and effective way to shut down the problem."

Exercise and nutrition are the supply pillars of the nerves. Lifestyle supports function, it doesn't control function. That's why one person eats organic, works out, doesn't drink or smoke and still gets cancer while another person drinks, smokes, eats bad food, never works out and you can't kill that person if you try. One very big piece of the puzzle has been overlooked for too long. If our nerve supply has been compromised, it doesn't matter what we do. Sickness will come.

The nervous system and immune system are hardwired and work together to keep your body functioning optimally. If your spine is out of alignment neural dysfunctions stress your body and cause hindrances within its perfect design. Chiropractic care removes interference in the central nervous system, which controls and coordinates all the functions of your body.

Once your spine is corrected your body can function correctly and heal itself wherever necessary.

In 1975, Ronald Pero, Ph.D., chief of cancer prevention research at New York's Preventive Medicine Institute and professor in Environmental Health at New York University published over 160 reports, making him an expert in individual susceptibility to various chronic diseases.

Pero recognized the relationship cancer-inducing agents had on the endocrine system, which is regulated by the nervous system. He began to see what chiropractors have been saying for years, the nervous system influences susceptibility to cancer and other diseases.

He gathered a lot of literature linking various kinds of spinal cord injuries to cancers and found that there was a significantly high rate of lymphomas and lymphatic leukemias. Pero began to consider chiropractic care as a means of reducing the risk of immune breakdown and disease. He tested his theory with a team of 107 people who had received long-term chiropractic care. The chiropractic patients were shown to have a 200% greater immune competence than people who had not received chiropractic care and a 400% greater immune competence than people with cancer or serious diseases.

Age isn't a factor when it comes to enjoying the benefits of spinal adjustments. Pero found no decline with the various age groups in the study demonstrating that the DNA repairing enzymes were just as present in long-term chiropractic senior groups as they were in the younger groups. The expert concluded, "Chiropractic may optimize whatever genetic abilities you have so that you can fully resist serious disease ... I have never seen a group other than this show a 200% increase over normal patients."

Eliminate the risk factors and build a healthier life for yourself. You don't have to feel powerless to this killer.

Why aren't medical doctors educating us on how spinal adjustments, exercise, diet, reducing toxins and stress are the first steps to defeating this enemy? Has the propaganda of Chemical Religion deceived even the professionals established to save lives?

## Could it Be That the Cure is Being Hidden?

When you ask the average person if they've ever been to a chiropractor most will say they have not. We've heard some express distrust and discrediting the profession as not being real doctors though they can't tell you the source of their fears. In reality, both M.D.s and Doctors of Chiropractic (D.C.s) spend just as much time and money on their studies. There's a shocking reason for this ignorant idea. I think you'll find it appalling.

Chiropractic isn't some weird, witch doctor practice someone recently came up with. It's been around since 1895 when a guy named Dr. D.D. Palmer adjusted the spine of a deaf janitor, Harvey Lillard, and his hearing returned. The good news traveled fast, and the profession grew. People either wanted to be a D.C. or they needed to see one. But this news of people getting well without medicine didn't make everyone as happy. In 1906, Dr. D.D. Palmer was the first of many chiropractors to be arrested. His only crime was making sick people well, or maybe for defunding the medical industry.

In 1918 the Spanish Flu killed 100 million people around the world and people turned to D.C.s for healing. In fact, for the first 70 years of chiropractic history, more people were seeing their D.C.s to treat their infectious diseases than for any other issue, including back pain. But by 1923 the war against the life-giving profession was getting bloody. Chiropractors were being thrown in jail for up to two years and many died there under work gangs meant to teach them a lesson. "Don't take our customers, or else."

The chiropractors persevered through the threats and mistreatment led by the medical industry because they believed in what they were doing. Every day they brought hope and healing to their patients. They knew they couldn't give up the fight, so in 1943 Dr. Leo Spears was able to build

the largest hospital in the U.S. all based on drugless chiropractic principles. Here countless cases deemed incurable by the M.D.s were made well.
Those with birth related injuries, polio, MS, POTS, those paralyzed from
trauma, war vets with broken backs and other crippling disabilities were
able to eventually walk, run and dance their way home from the hospital.

By the early 1960's chiropractic schools were popping up everywhere
because so many students wanted to spend their lives like the heroes they
had admired, while the students enrolling in medical school were declining. This infuriated some people in high places who feared losing their
power, so an evil plan was devised.

In 1962 the Iowa American Medical Association (IAMA) made it their
mission to contain and eliminate the chiropractic profession. Their plan
consisted of six steps.

1. Prevent D.C.s from seeing patients with work injuries.

2. Insurance should not cover chiropractic care.

3. Block D.C.s from having hospital privileges.

4. Discourage students from going to chiropractic school.

5. Encourage complaints of chiropractors whenever possible.

6. KEEP THE PLAN SECRET FROM THE PUBLIC

A year after the plan was set in motion, the American Medical Association
(AMA) joined forces and formed the "Committee on Quackery," also
known as the Committee to Get Rid of Chiropractic. Their mission was to:

1. Disseminate negative information about chiropractic to media,
   medical schools and the public.

2. Rid all positive information about chiropractic from the public
   and M.D.s.

3.  Put out of business M.D.s who associate with chiropractors.

Are you beginning to see how the medical profession isn't in business to find a cure? People were getting well. Instead of joining forces with the doctors who were delivering healing the AMA set itself against chiropractic and even stooped to deceiving the public and M.D.s, who actually cared for patients. Their propaganda began to work, and they deemed chiropractic as an "unscientific cult" in order to discredit it in their bylaws, Principle #3, which says, "A medical doctor cannot associate with an unscientific cult."

The chiropractic profession would've been extinct forever had it not been for the brave doctors like Chester Wilks, along with three other chiropractors, who faced the powerful bully with a lawsuit against the AMA, the American College of Surgeons, the American College of Physicians and the Joint Commission on Accreditation of Hospitals. The fight was long and expensive, beginning in 1976; but in 1981 the court battle to save chiropractic was lost. Wilks refused to give up and won on appeal in 1983, to which the superpower countered in multiple appeals. The United States Supreme Court, who was visually angry for the injustice inflicted upon Wilks and the rest of the chiropractic community, convicted all defendants of conspiracy to eliminate and constrain the practice of chiropractic, forbidding them from further appeals in 1992.

## Chemo the Cure That Kills

The medical organizations may have lost the battle, but they still managed to accomplish their mission to contain the chiropractic profession through false information, fear tactics against patients and by inhibiting the submission of chiropractic care to insurance companies.

Insurance companies are in deep with the Chemical Religion and refuse to pay for anything preventative or nonmedical. People are scared of being punished with debilitating bills if they refuse the treatments recommended by their M.D. What they don't realize is how inexpensive true health is in comparison to the never-ending roller coaster chemical patients suffer. They hop on that ride seeking answers for one illness, and may stabilize it for a moment, only to throw up their arms in terror again when that medicine jerks them down another scary diagnosis.

In desperation, cancer patients don't ask questions when the doctor orders chemotherapy. They know it means they will lose their hair. They've heard how sick chemotherapy makes patients who are battling for their lives and how their quality of life is sometimes so depressing they'd rather die than keep fighting. They have their reservations, but they don't see any other options, because the only hope a medical doctor can offer is a killer.

Many become martyrs for their faith in the Chemical Religion—and for what? Chemotherapy fails 98% of its patients. When compared to doing nothing at all, doing nothing beat chemo as a better option!

Once convinced, a cancer patient will likely undergo invasive testing. Chemo sensitivity testing requires extracting cells from a cancerous tumor. The cancer is tested with different chemotherapies to see which drug will successfully beat it. This may be all right if it had a redeeming value, but it doesn't! Chemo sensitivity testing not only endangers the patient by possibly changing a pre-malignant tissue to a malignant one, but it changes the microenvironment of that tissue, thus changing the gene expression that's being assessed. It's surprising that oncology has overlooked the science of tumors called *inflammatory oncotaxis* that explains why cutting into a tumor is a bad idea.

Our body's natural first response to a grouping of sick cells is to protect us by encapsulating it. When we stab it, the cancer can spread, causing secondary tumors. Once exposed, the tumor changes. The cells being tested with chemo no longer resemble the tumor; therefore, whatever drug may work on the cells that have been removed won't necessarily work on the tumor.

So begins a patient's battle to stay alive through the treatment that is literally attacking every cell in their body. Chemo drugs such as imatinib, known under the brand Gleevec, used for leukemia and sunitinib in the brand Sutent, and also used for gastrointestinal tumors, may initially reduce tumor size but soon cause tumors to come back aggressively stronger and larger than before.

Other drugs meant to block nutrients and oxygen from tumors are often paired with chemotherapy, making for a bigger disaster. When researchers induced anti-angiogenesis into mice, it seemed like the pharmaceutical had a win seeing a 30% decrease in the volume of the tumor over 25 days. The "win" soon proved to be another *fail* by Rx companies when the tumors that had moved to the lungs tripled.

In the past, kings would have their chef try the food first before consuming it. If the chef refused, royalty might wonder if they were in danger of being poisoned. In today's world of medicine, a survey of those writing out prescriptions was conducted, and over 88% of doctors confessed that if they were terminally ill, they would rather die naturally than take what they're recommending to their patients. Why would they encourage a treatment they wouldn't consider for themselves?

*The Journal of the American Medical Association* reported that as much as 75% of the average oncologist's earnings come from in-office chemotherapy drug sells. The mark-up alone in many offices is arguably criminal. "What we found in the marketplace is that over one quarter of the medical centers that provide cancer services are charging more than 5.1 times the Medicare allowable amount, and in some cases the centers are charging more than 15 times the Medicare allowable amount," stated Martin Makary, M.D., MPH, a cancer surgeon at Johns Hopkins Hospital and lead author of the study published in the *American Journal of Managed Care,* which examined the price of care at more than 3,200 hospitals in all 50 states.

Doctors have also received illegal kickbacks from pharmaceutical companies for asserting their products. AstraZeneca, Inc. had to pay $280 million in civil penalties and $63 million in criminal penalties to the federal government for incentivizing M.D.s promoting their prostate cancer drug.

That's not the only conflict of interest between some oncologists and pharmaceutical companies. Chemo is sold by oncologists who have become among the highest paid specialists in medicine. Some make as much as two-thirds their income from chemo drugs. Oncologists buy these drugs direct at wholesale prices, then they mark them up and bill the insurance companies. Some chemotherapy drugs have a higher profit margin than others. We find it alarming when a doctor is recommending drugs based on personal gain verses their patients' well-being.

Oncologists who care more about their patients than their bottom line are still prescribing unfounded cancer treatments simply because hospitals and doctors are reimbursed for carrying out the standardized cancer procedures. Even if a medical doctor wanted to recommend an alternative treatment, insurance companies will only pay for what they are told by Big Pharma works, no matter how many times it fails. Doctors who do not comply are in danger of losing their license.

The doctors are wise to avoid such treatments for themselves. *The Lancet Oncology* published a study that revealed chemotherapy treatments kill up to 50% of cancer patients in some hospitals.

Long-time advocate against orthodox cancer treatment, the late Dr. Hardin B. Jones Professor of Medical Physics and Physiology at Berkeley, California, was published in the New York Academy of Science as saying, "People who refused chemotherapy treatment live on average 12 ½ years longer than people who are undergoing chemotherapy. Those who accepted other kinds of treatment lived an average of only 3 years. Beyond the shadow of a doubt, radical surgery on cancer patients does more harm than good."

The evidence against the standard cancer treatments is being ignored. Chemotherapy causes cancer. It's printed right on the chemo drug warning labels! When examining the effects of chemotherapy on tissue removed from men with prostate cancer there's strong evidence of DNA damage. Scientists who performed the research say that a protein called WNT16B is created from chemo treatment, and it boosts cancer cell survival. They believe it's the reason that chemotherapy actually ends lives more quickly.

## The Early Detection Scam

Whenever we hear a phrase repeated regularly until it becomes an end all argument catch phrase we have to wonder if it's propaganda. Phrases like, "the benefits outweigh the risks," and "we're in this together" are repeated until they're no longer questioned. Compliance becomes the only option in the heads of those who have not been better informed. So, when we hear all this talk about "early detection" around cancer survival that's making women without cancer run to the oncologist to have their breasts removed, we're skeptical, to say the least.

Is all this screening necessary or is it putting healthy people at risk? One study with 1,087 individuals participating in a cancer screening trial who received a battery of tests for prostate, ovarian, colorectal and lung cancer exposed that 43% had at least one false positive test result. This study, published in an issue of Cancer Epidemiology Biomarkers & Prevention, is concerning when we consider the emotional trauma a family experiences when told they have a life-threatening disease. It also makes us wonder how many have received treatment unnecessarily.

We'll go into more depth in chapter 10 about the dangers of radiation from medical equipment such as ultrasounds, but mammograms expose women to regular treatments of radiation as well. We're trying to understand the logic in preventing cancer through "early detection" by exposing patients to cancer causing radiation. Like so much of medicine, it doesn't make sense.

Seeking the good and bad effects of breast cancer screening, researchers from the Nordic Cochrane Center in Demark reviewed seven breast cancer screening programs that included 500,000 women. For every 2,000 women who received mammograms over a 10-year period, only one would have her life prolonged, but ten would be harmed.

The case against mammograms continues to build as more studies emerge. It increases a woman's risk of developing breast cancer by as much as 3% in each breast a year by exposing the breast cells to radiation and triggering breast cancer. The numbers suggest that Komen's investment in women's mammograms may actually be doing them more harm than good.

Many mammograms have been found to be mis-calibrated. The radiation emitted exceeds what is estimated to be safe. Women are being scared into getting tested with the "early detection" propaganda but when they begin getting routine mammograms at age 40, twenty years later all that radiation has them at serious risk of developing breast cancer because of the mammograms.

Safe detection has been discovered. It comes inexpensively and with zero risks, but it's unlikely to gain popularity because it doesn't make money. A simple saliva test can do the trick thanks to researchers from the University of Texas Health Science Center in Houston who discovered that women with breast cancer carry different proteins than women with no cancer.

Health can be found, but not usually in the places our society has come to trust. Are you willing to look for answers from sources that have not been spreading lies?

Why do some people distrust chiropractors? For the same reason that there's still no cure declared for cancer and other "incurable" diseases. The people behind the Chemical Religion have hidden the truth and have indoctrinated us with their lies. Their greed and lust for power have affected us all, but now that we know the truth, we are set free; free to stop spending money on healthcare that doesn't cure the disease; free to stop running marathons that fund a billion-dollar industry: and free to defund cancer and spread the news that there is a cure.

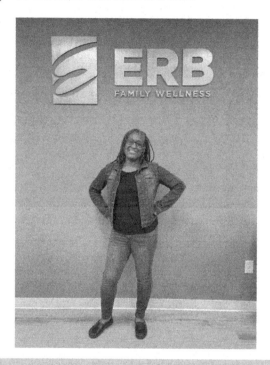

I was severely depressed. I had severe pain in my neck and shoulder. It was indescribable. I had just received a breast cancer diagnosis after discovering a lump, later to be identified as a tumor. I was scared for my life. I didn't know what was going to happen. I was just hurting from the inside out.

A friend of mine told me about Dr. Erb and said I should really get there and check him out. I was a little skeptical, really not sure what to expect. I had been to other places similar, and I was like, "No, I'm not going." But I went. And when I got there, when I opened the door, there was hope like I've never seen before. There was a shift from the front door to the back door.

I walked in, I did the testing, [metabolic, thermography, x-rays]. I talked, which I wasn't doing much of. I was able to see changes immediately. I got my energy back; I got my strength back. I came alive again! I was literally dying on the inside and I woke up. I came alive.

The pain, something I had been struggling with for years, was gone. The tumor was shrinking. I did some labs and with the results I had no cancer in my body. So that was a pure miracle. I was able to not only get myself help, but I got my whole family help. Everybody is changed radically as a result of being at Erb Family Wellness. They have the answers that you are looking for.

I'm cancer free, free from depression, and continue to maintain a chemical free and healthy lifestyle. – Mia Gray

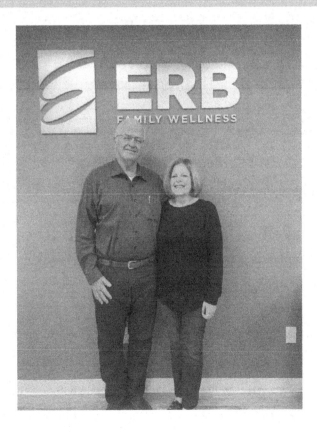

My wife Pam has been a patient of Erb Family Wellness for five years. Her health has benefitted a lot from the program the Erb Family Wellness outlined for her.

When my health issues became worse, it was only natural for me to also become a patient of Erb Family Wellness.

Prior to becoming a patient of the Erb Family Wellness, I had three issues:

- Prostate cancer that was confirmed with a biopsy and an elevated PSA test.

- A stiff neck that made it difficult to turn my head.

- Severe left knee pain from an injury.

After becoming a patient at Erb Family Wellness, a set of tests were given to address areas that needed attention:

- Thermography

- Metabolic Test

- X-ray

These tests were reviewed by Drs. David and Kimberly Erb, and they prescribed a plan that started me on a road to recovery.

The following plan was prescribed:

- A specific meal plan that includes delicious healthy recipes.

- Home rehab exercises, interval training and walking.

- Being adjusted in the Erb Wellness center with special emphasis on spinal correction including neck, back and left knee adjustments.

- Supplements

- Metabolic retest

- Conclusion after one year:

- PSA level was lowered from a 4.65 to a 3.91

- Stiff neck was drastically reduced. I used to have issues from a stiff neck looking over my shoulder while merging onto a freeway or behind me when operating our farm tractor.

- Left knee is completely free of pain and strength is getting stronger every week.

- Normalized blood pressure allowing me to eliminate prescription medication.

- Immune system vastly improved. I have been free of flu and colds for a year.

In closing, my wife and I appreciate the Erb's and their Christian faith. Dr. David always starts each session with a scripture quotation and devotion.

My wife and I have three generations of family as patients at the Erb Family Wellness. This includes our daughter, grandson and Pam and me. – Ralph and Pam Todd

# CHAPTER 6
# ARE YOU CREATING
# THE PERFECT STORM?

"No one hates his own body but feeds and cares for it, just as
Christ cares for the church." Ephesians 5:29 NLT

If you live anywhere from Texas to southern Minnesota you've experienced having your TV or radio station interrupted announcing a Severe Thunderstorm WATCH. Meteorologists are watching the weather 24/7 for elements that could create destructive thunderstorms. When they see conditions come together, they break into a broadcast and issue an alert.

Storms are created when an upward center of low pressure develops within a system of high pressure. An upward current of air (called an updraft) forms when warm, moist air meets cold temperatures. These opposing forces can create winds resulting in the formation of storm clouds, lightning, high winds and hail.

We may not be able to control the weather, but our actions can indirectly influence where thunderstorms form. Increased temperatures in and around cities due to the urban heat island effect can trigger thunderstorms in areas that wouldn't typically suffer a storm. High-pressure areas move and grow. As they do, a low-pressure area, the storm, will shift directions and take *the path of least resistance* around the high-pressure system.

The devastation caused by storms is immeasurable. Fires, flash floods, tornadoes and hail can be deadly and expensive. The aftermath is often irreparable. If we could protect our homes from their terror, we would certainly take whatever precautions necessary. But there's another kind of storm brewing, one for which we have more power to resist.

Just like there are elements that come together in our atmosphere to wreak havoc on our land in low pressure areas; if we're not willing to endure some high pressure as we resist going with the flow of the Chemical Religion, we're allowing the elements to create the perfect storm within our body. This storm's destruction takes many forms, but it's best known as autoimmunity.

We're issuing a Severe Thunderstorm WATCH. We see the conditions for which a storm could form and are sending out a warning to be watchful and vigilant.

The elements creating a perfect storm within our body include:

- Vaccinations
- GMOs
- Chemical exposures
- Food additives
- Rx drugs
- Antibiotics
- Decreased nerve supply
- EMFs (Electromagnetic fields)

Like the weather, we may not be able to completely avoid all of these factors, but we can take actions to resist them and their deadly results.

## What is Autoimmune Disease?

A raging storm began in 1989 when huge amounts of mercury and other metals began to be injected through vaccines. The storms raged within our body against our own body. Autoimmune disease is a disease in which the body produces antibodies that attack its own tissues leading to the deterioration and in some cases to the destruction of such tissue. It now doubles the number of people who have cancer.

When we were growing up, peanut allergies were unheard of. Now there are nut-free tables set aside at school cafeterias for kids who could potentially die from exposure. Some have died. One teenage girl kissed her boyfriend after he had consumed a peanut butter sandwich and the allergic reaction took her life. Parents who have children with severe allergies often suffer from anxiety as they have to entrust them to schools and daycare. This once obscure disease has become an epidemic. But how?

Autoimmune disease, also known as *"The Western Disease,"* affects 24 million Americans, costing $591 million in research and treatment a year.

- Mayo Clinic researchers say rising rates of lupus are the result of an increased exposure to environmental triggers of some unknown origin.

- Type 1 Diabetes researchers insist the rapid rise cannot be explained by better diagnostics or a rise in genetic factors, but rather a change in environmental circumstances.

- 9.8 million women are afflicted with one of the seven most common autoimmune diseases.

With nearly 100 autoimmune diseases such as Type 1 Diabetes, Celiac, Psoriasis, Hashimotos, Fibromyalgia, Crohn's, Chronic Fatigue Syndrome and Rheumatoid Arthritis (to name a few), this storm raging against our own bodies has medical doctors scratching their heads without any answers.

Maybe take another pill to combat the symptoms, then yet another to combat those symptoms? Is autoimmune disease caused by a drug deficiency? We think not.

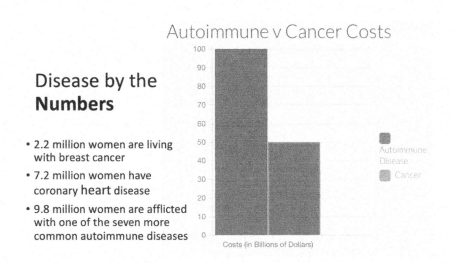

How is Autoimmune Disease Incurred?

Our baptism of chemicals and toxins begin at birth. We're immediately vaccinated and injected with more toxins when we're taken to routine well-baby checkups. From the beginning we are met with formulas loaded with GMOs, more well-baby stabbings, school lunches loaded with the GMOs or convenience bagged lunches, hand sanitizers in every classroom, lack of exercise inhibiting our oxygen intake, cell phone EMFs, a stressful fast-paced lifestyle, and over-the-counter meds. We're completely polluting our body! Is it any wonder why our body is turning on itself with these diseases?

- SLE (Lupus)- Tissues, Joints, Skin, Cartilage
- Multiple Sclerosis- Myelin
- Parkinson's- Brain
- Vitiligo - Skin pigment cells
- Autoimmune Hepatitis- Liver
- Sjogren's- Glands

- Alopecia- Hair follicles
- Hemolytic Anemia- Red Blood Cells

EMF radiation is a strong force that opposes our immune system. It's an invisible, silent poison we are all ingesting day and night. When it meets other opposing forces fighting our immune system, a perfect storm can form. It may be an autoimmune disease, or it could be among a long list of other serious issues. (We've included a more extensive list in the Appendix.)

Like currents of wind these subtle energies constantly swirl in and around our bodies, though we are usually unaware of them. EMFs are energy waves with frequencies below 300 hertz or cycles per second. The electromagnetic fields we encounter daily come from everyday things such as power lines, radar and microwave towers, television and computer screens, motors, fluorescent lights, microwave ovens, cell phones, electric blankets, house wiring, and hundreds of other common electrical devices. They are inescapable in today's world, and frequent exposure can cause biological health effects.

EMF radiation suppresses our immune system, making it more difficult for our body to fight viruses, bacteria, molds and whatever else might attack our health. Research indicates EMF radiation may be creating antibiotic-resistant pathogens. We're beginning to see that they may be reducing good bacteria and increasing bad bacteria. Some doctors have noticed that their patients are not recovering. They are beginning to attribute this to an electromagnetic field immunosuppressant impact that disables our immune response.

A pilot study published in *Immunology Research* recruited 64 patients with various autoimmune diagnoses such as systematic lupus erythematosus, rheumatoid arthritis, multiple sclerosis, Sjogren's syndrome, and celiac disease. The researchers blocked exposure to EMFs in the patients, resulting in the significant relief of symptoms for 90% of patients. For four hours at night and four hours during the day, subjects wore shielded clothing that was partially capable of blocking penetration of microwave EMF. This research group concluded that patients with autoimmune disorders were noticeably susceptible to EMFs at levels common in work and home environments. Their observations led them to consider that EMFs may be a contributing factor to the process the autoimmune disease develops and progresses.

In Chapter 13 we will explain how you can resist the powerful force of EMFs and avoid the perfect storm that leads to autoimmune disease, but first we want to share how vaccinations also swirl together with EMFs and other immune opposing forces to cause our body to war against itself.

Adjuvants are substances put into vaccines to stimulate stronger immune responses. Other toxic ingredients are also included in the potion, such as:

- Excipients/preservatives lab altered viruses and bacteria
- Aluminum
- Mercury
- Formaldehyde
- Phenoxyethanol
- Glutaraldehyde
- Sodium borate
- Sodium chloride
- Ethylene glycol (antifreeze)
- Monosodium glutamate (MSG)
- Hydrochloric acid
- Hydrogen peroxide
- Lactose
- Gelatin
- Sorbitol and other unidentified contaminants
- Egg albumin
- Yeast protein
- Antibiotics
- Phenol (carbolic acid)
- Borax (ant killer)
- Sodium acetate
- Dye
- Acetone (nail polish remover)
- Bovine and human serum albumin
- Glycerol
- Polysorbate 80/20
- Latex

When you review the ingredients, it looks like a couple of kids went through their parents' cabinets and threw a bunch of stuff together to see what would happen. Somehow, scientists decided that this toxic combination that mixed in adjuvants would manipulate our immune system (to respond more aggressively to diseases) would be a safe and effective aid. But is heightening and stimulating our natural immune response a good thing, or is it messing with God's design and making us sick?

Researchers at the University of Virginia Health System's Division of Asthma & Immunology report that an era of food allergies, which began with the post-millennial generation, might be a response to vaccines containing the adjuvant alum (aluminum hydroxide, potassium aluminum sulfate), a known trigger for allergic traits.

In a study out of Japan, scientists took mice that were naturally unlikely to develop autoimmunity and showed that with repeated overstimulation from vaccines on an individual's immune system, every individual will develop autoimmunity disorders. We are experiencing an epidemic of autoimmune disease because we're subjecting ourselves to these shots!

## 1960 — 5

Polio
Smallpox
DPT*

*3-dose vaccines:
- DPT/DTaP: diphtheria, tetanus, pertussis
- MMR: measles, mumps, rubella

## 1983 — 24

DPT* (2 mos.)
OPV (2 mos.)
DPT* (4 mos.)
OPV (4 mos.)
DPT* (6 mos.)
MMR* (15 mos.)
DPT* (18 mos.)
OPV (18 mos.)
DPT* (4 yrs.)
OPV (4 yrs.)
Td (15 yrs.)

### 1986—Liability Shield

Vaccine makers were granted 100% immunity from liability under the 1986 National Childhood Vaccine Injury Act. Parents/consumers cannot sue vaccine companies when their products injure. Since then, the childhood vaccine schedule has significantly increased. There are now hundreds of new vaccines in development.

## 2019** — 74

Influenza (pregnancy)
DTap* (pregnancy)
Hep B (birth)
Hep B (2 mos.)
Rotavirus (2 mos.)
DTap* (2 mos.)
HIB (2 mos.)
PCV (2 mos.)
IPV (2 mos.)
Rotavirus (4 mos.)
DTap* (4 mos.)
HIB (4 mos.)
PCV (4 mos.)
IPV (4 mos.)
Hep B (6 mos.)
Rotavirus (6 mos.)
DTap* (6 mos.)
HIB (6 mos.)
PCV (6 mos.)
IPV (6 mos.)
Influenza (6 mos.)
Influenza (7 mos.)
HIB (12 mos.)
PCV (12 mos.)
MMR* (12 mos.)
Varicella (12 mos.)
Hep A (12 mos.)
DTap* (18 mos.)

Influenza (18 mos.)
Hep A (18 mos.)
Influenza (30 mos.)
Influenza (42 mos.)
DTaP* (4 yrs.)
IPV (4 yrs.)
MMR* (4 yrs.)
Varicella (4 yrs.)
Influenza (5 yrs.)
Influenza (6 yrs.)
Influenza (7 yrs.)
Influenza (8 yrs.)
Influenza (9 yrs.)
HPV (9 yrs.)
Influenza (10 yrs.)
HPV (10 yrs.)
Influenza (11 yrs.)
HPV (11 yrs.)
DTap* (12 yrs.)
Influenza (12 yrs.)
Meningococcal (12 yrs.)
Influenza (13 yrs.)
Influenza (14 yrs.)
Influenza (15 yrs.)
Influenza (16 yrs.)
Meningococcal (16 yrs.)
Influenza (17 yrs.)
Influenza (18 yrs.)

**CDC current recommended vaccine schedule

## CDC Recommended Childhood Vaccine Schedule: 1986 vs 2019

| 1986 ⇒ | 12 shots / 25 antigens / 8 diseases | 2019 ⇒ | 54 shots / 70 antigens / 16 diseases |
|---|---|---|---|
| DTP (2 Months) | MMR (15 Months) DTP (4 Years) | Hep B (1 day) | Influenza (7 Months) Influenza (5 years) |
| Polio (2 Months) | DTP (18 Months) Polio (4 Years) | Hep B (1 Month) | MMR (12 Months) Influenza (6 Years) |
| DTP (4 Months) | Polio (18 Months) Td (14 Years) | DTaP (2 Months) | Varicella (12 Months) Influenza (7 Years) |
| Polio (4 Months) | Hib (2 Years) | Polio (2 Months) | Hib (12 Months) Influenza (8 Years) |
| DTP (6 Months) | | Hib (2 Months) | Hep A (12 Months) Influenza (9 Years) |
| | | PCV 13 (2 Months) | PCV 13 (12 Months) Influenza (10 Years) |
| | | Rotavirus (2 Months) | DTaP (15 Months) HPV (11 Years) |
| | | DTaP (4 Months) | Hep A (18 Months) Meningococcal ACWY (11 Years) |
| | | Polio (4 Months) | Influenza (18 Months) |
| | | Hib (4 Months) | Influenza (2 Years) Tdap (11 Years) |
| | | PCV 13 (4 Months) | Influenza (3 Years) Influenza (11 Years) |
| | | Rotavirus (4 Months) | Influenza (4 years) HPV (11.5 Years) |
| | | DTaP (6 Months) | DTaP (4 Years) Influenza (12 years) |
| | | Polio (6 Months) | MMR (4 Years) Influenza (13 Years) |
| | | Hep B (6 months) | Polio (4 Years) Influenza (14 Years) |
| | | Hib (6 Months) | Varicella (4 Years) Influenza (15 Years) |
| | | PCV 13 (6 Months) | Meningococcal ACWY (16 Years) |
| | | Rotavirus (6 Months) | Influenza (16 Years) |
| | | Influenza (6 Months) | Influenza (17 Years) |
| | | | Influenza (18 years) |

Children's Health Defense

You can see from these charts how many more injections children today are inflicted with in comparison to when we were kids. Most parents who grew up with vaccinations think, "We turned out fine, our kids won't be harmed either." But when we realize that the overabundance of poison children's immune systems are being subjected to, it defies comparison. Our bodies are created to heal and overcome, but eventually they become overrun with vaccines, and that is what we are seeing today. It has created the perfect storm—and autoimmune disease is the consequence.

Those vaccinated increase their susceptibility for the following:

- Asthma increased 4.6 times

- Eczema, allergic rashes increased 2.5 times

- Chronic otitis (ear issues) increased 3 times

- Recurrent tonsillitis increased 3.3 times

- Sudden infant death increased 4 times

- Hyperactivity increased 9.4 times

**There is no path to better health through better chemistry**! "Medical practice has neither philosophy nor common sense to recommend it. In sickness the body is already loaded with impurities. By taking drugs – medicines more impurities are added, thereby the case is further embarrassed and harder to cure" said Elmer Lee, M.D., past Vice President of the Academy of Medicine. Vaccinations are not the cure. They are often the cause.

- "The results of suppressing measles and other infectious diseases [by vaccinations] are cancer and other auto-immune and chronic diseases." Scheibner V. *Immunization: The Medical Assault on the Immune System*. Blackheath, Australia: Author, 1993; xxii.

- Harris Coulter, Ph.D. (medical historian) revealed childhood immunizations to be causing a low-grade encephalitis in about 15-20% of all infants.

- A study in *Lancet* reported that Crohn's disease and ulcerative colitis were far more prevalent in vaccinated individuals than non-vaccinated.

Glyphosate is another dark cloud playing a part in the autoimmune storm, including celiac disease, which affects the small intestine. Some researchers have concluded that glyphosate is possibly the most important factor in the development of the multiple chronic diseases and conditions that have become prevalent in Westernized societies. The herbicide causes extreme disruption of microbes' functions and lifecycles. What's worse, glyphosate preferentially affects beneficial bacteria, allowing pathogens to overgrow. Avoid foods that are not organic and non-GMO, or you will likely be consuming glyphosate.

Prescription drug use is another element in this perfect storm our culture is creating. Robert Henderson, M.D. cautions, "Every drug increases and complicates the patients' condition." For example:

- Antibiotics wipes out the bacteria ecosystem, thins gut lining, leads to leaky gut and poor absorption.

- NSAIDS (pain relievers such as aspirin and ibuprofin) cause damage and bleeding in the GI tract, can cause inflammation response, immune response combined with GMOs and sugars. They lead to autoimmune disease.

- Antidepressants wreck our serotonin system (90% of serotonin is made in the gut).

- Blood pressure meds, the majority made from synthesized snake venom from South America, are obviously bad for your gut when swallowed, and it damages the lungs, causing a chronic cough.

Glyphosate, food additives, and increased consumption of processed foods combined with constant increasing mandatory vaccines have led to hyper-stimulated immune systems and the outbreak of mental illness in children like never seen before! One in 28 boys have autism, 50% of children now have a chronic disease and 21% of all U.S. children are developmentally disabled.

Every chemical forces the body to use up precious resources in order to detox and heal. Combine that reaction with decreased nerve supply, and you have all the elements to create the perfect storm.

The spine has been overlooked for too long for the part it plays in our overall health. Even for a perfectly curved spine, receiving regular adjustments are beneficial providing more immunity power than drinking vitamin C to knock out colds and viruses. When a spine is misaligned, it can lead to autoimmune diseases, chronic diseases, and all kinds of other health issues. If you experience any of the symptoms below, consider them warning signs for a spine in danger of subluxation and keep reading. (We'll show you how to get the help you need in Chapter 13.)

- Hormone Issues
- Poor digestion / Skin Issues
- Lower back pain
- Sciatica
- Allergies / Asthma / Sinus / Ear issues
- Poor sleep
- Lowered Immunity
- Fatigue
- High Blood Pressure
- Headaches
- Neck pain

- Numbness / pain in arms, legs, feet

## How Do We Resist?

Be the resistance so the storm doesn't land in your life. We live in a culture brainwashed by the Chemical Religion. Going against the flow isn't easy, but it's the only way to protect our homes from the diseases plaguing those who follow blindly.

Resistance begins with repentance (or *changing direction*). Resist and turn away from consuming the kinds of toxic foods and products that we discussed in Chapters Two and Three. Resist a sedentary lifestyle and turn to exercise instead. Resist the propaganda that spine health isn't covered by insurance and is therefore unnecessary. Chiropractic visits are the most effective doctor's visits you can have. A healthy spine is insurance for your organs. It protects the nerve supply being carried to each one.

Action Steps:

- Eliminate Vaccines- get waivers from your state (see Chapter 1, 13)
- Non-GMO foods- Certified Organic (see Chapter 2)
- Metabolix Testing (see Chapter 13)
- 14-day GI Reboot Plan (see Chapter 13)
- Most advanced eating diet (see Chapter 13)
- Minimize your chemical exposures (see Chapter 2, 3, and Appendix)
- Protect yourself from EMFs (see Chapter 13 and Appendix)
- Nerve Supply (see Chapter 13)

Abraham Lincoln was right when he said, "A house divided against itself cannot stand." Autoimmunity is the storm of the body turning against itself. It starts in the grocery store and in the kind of healthcare we choose. Every day we make a decision to go with the flow, or to resist. Every day we can choose to be healthy and take cover from the storm or choose to do what everyone else is doing until we get a bad report, a Severe Thunderstorm WARNING. The storm doesn't reach our own flesh until we have ignored the Severe Thunderstorm WATCH. We decide.

We can help you take cover. M.D.s diagnose autoimmune diseases with an incurable prognosis, but we've seen all kinds of "incurable" diseases healed.

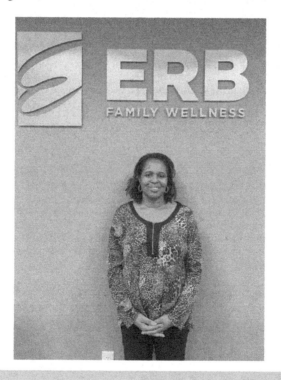

They have changed my life!!! I was diagnosed with multiple sclerosis when I was 29 years old. It was 1999 and I was a new lawyer ready to take off with my career. I started tremoring and having symptoms. I have never been one to accept sickness. I believed in the power of prayer and in a God who heals. I prayed, "I can't do this. What are we going to do

Lord?" I like to move and be outdoors! I like to dance! Multiple sclerosis would take those things away from me.

I was trying to figure out how to get well when I saw Dr. Kimberly at Wingstop in 2007. She invited me to the office, and I started care. I was completely relieved from *all* my symptoms. I have never had any meds for this disease. I still work. I am still high energy. I am still practicing law. And I still dance! I am able to do all this because I am well.

Over the years I have stayed well. My family is full of cancer and heart disease. Everyone is on meds on both sides. I don't have any of that. I am 51 years old. My younger sister is on all kind of meds. She and I went to see my mother who was 75 and getting knee replacement surgery. I was the only one strong enough to really care for mom. My sister did her best, but she isn't well either.

I have remained under the care of the Erbs for all these years. It is preventative health care and maintenance for my body. I recently went to an Erb Family Wellness Makeover seminar where they talked about the benefits of intermittent fasting. I have lost 37 pounds since I began this practice! My appetites have changed. I don't have the cravings I use to experience. Eating good, healthy foods curb my appetite because it nourishes my body with what it needs. I could go on and on in sharing how Erb Family Wellness has impacted my health. I experienced the effects of shedding from my boyfriend after he got the Covid vaccine. The Erbs recommended more adjustments, zinc, vitamin D and C. I also did the hyperbaric chamber two times. After the second time I had so much energy and felt better. I even cleaned up my whole house. That hyperbaric is like a magic time machine! I could barely walk when I got in. The second visit got me back into my life. It's now a regular part of my wellness plan.

I have not had a relapse of MS in 10 years. I don't see the MDs because they don't have anything that can heal me.

We are so blessed to have Dr. David and Dr. Kimberly speaking into our lives. - Toni McCarty

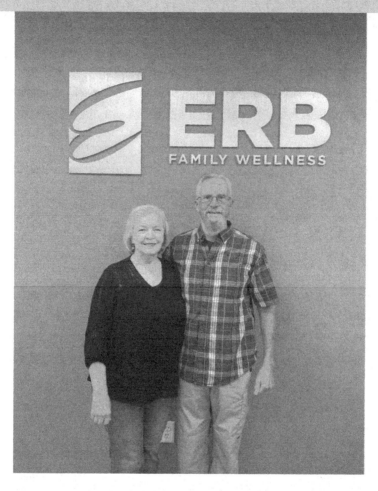

We came to Erb Family Wellness about 12 years ago when Bonnie was experiencing significant symptoms and facing gall bladder surgery. I thought I was in pretty good health, but I was getting bronchitis and pneumonia every winter.

At our initial consultation with Dr. Dave, we BOTH started care and began our journey of implementing the five practices for better health. We started getting our spines adjusted, changed our diet according to the plan they laid out for us, and even changed how we exercise. We've had fantastic results. Bonnie's symptoms resolved, her surgery never happened, and we haven't had bronchitis or pneumonia in a decade!

Metabolic testing showed that I had leaky gut and toxicity. This condition was manifesting itself with skin problems like eczema. More dietary and supplementation changes resulted in healing in my gut and clearing of my skin. Removal of mercury fillings also were key to resolving the skin issues.

We were ready for Corona! I had Covid 19 in February of 2020 and felt awful for a week or so but believe that my history with the better health practices the Erbs taught me equipped my body to defeat the virus! Bonnie got it in November 2021 and had an even easier time with it. We are thankful to not be in fear of this virus!

We are far healthier than we were a decade ago when we started this journey and have no regrets. We remain active in our church and community and look forward to what God has for us each new day. – Ed and Bonnie Ouellette

# CHAPTER 7
# MAYBE IT'S NOT ALL IN YOUR HEAD

"A cheerful heart is good medicine, but a crushed
spirit dries up the bones."

Proverbs 17:22 NIV

We live in a fast-food culture. We don't even want to get out of our car
to feed ourselves. We don't like to be inconvenienced by our natural yet
uncomfortable human experiences such as hunger, but God forbid we
experience pain in this fallen world. Not to worry, the Chemical Religion
has a pill for that too. If we're sad, we must suffer from depression. If we're
shy, we must have social anxiety. There are new "diseases" being manufactured by pharmaceutical companies for every human emotion or behavior
for which man is inflicted.

## Are Depression and Mental Illness Chemical Imbalances
## or Propaganda?

Our brain can change based on our environment. Stress, sleep patterns and pain are a few things that effect the way we think, feel and the choices we make. Much of the psychiatric field has put too much emphasis on the biology of the brain while ignoring the impact of what a person has been through.

The chemical imbalance *theory* has been pushed by the Diagnostic and Statistical Manual of Mental Disorders, Fifth Edition (DSM-5). It's basically the psychiatric bible. Its content comes from a committee influenced by Big Pharma to diagnose mental illnesses for which they've concocted money-making pills. They can't make money from methods that actually *help* patients to deal with life's disappointing circumstances. Instead, they would rather serve up a snack to mask symptoms and produce an altered state similar to tranquilizers, which numb normal biological functions.

Propaganda and marketing have played a huge roll in changing what we believe about mental health. In the 1960's, Merck bought and distributed to psychiatrists tens of thousands of copies of books promoting the diagnosis of depression. SmithKline Beecham, Eli Lilly, Upjohn Pharmaceuticals and others used similar tactics in an effort to push their agenda making the chemical imbalance theory mainstream. Some drug companies influenced the media into giving these drugs terms such as "Wonder Drug" (*Time*, 1954), making them appealing to the general public.

If this chemical imbalance theory which includes drug therapy is valid, then why was there still nearly 45,000 suicides (or more) that occur annually in the United States? Suicide is among the top 10 leading causes of death! This crisis isn't getting better: according to the CDC, in half of the states in our country, suicide increased by more than 30% among people ages 10 and older from a 1999-2001 study to a study in 2014-2016.

## Do Antidepressants Cause Brain Damage?

Dr. Caroline Leaf is a communication pathologist and cognitive neuroscientist with a master's and PhD in Communication Pathology and a BSc in Logopaedics, specializing in cognitive and metacognitive neuropsychology. She says, "Even if someone feels that these psychoactive substances do help them, they are not correcting an underlying chemical imbalance in their brain, and potentially creating neurological imbalances that were not there to begin with. These drugs start changing our neurochemistry within the **first dose**." (Emphasis added)

Even the drug companies have been forced to admit that psychotropic drugs increase risk of suicide! It just doesn't make sense that something that's known to cause suicide to a level that the FDA couldn't ignore would be prescribed to patients already at risk.

Below is the FDA-mandated medication guide for Paxil and other antidepressants:

- Attempts to commit suicide
- Acting on dangerous impulses
- Acting aggressive or violent
- New or worse anxiety or panic attacks
- An increase in activity or talking more than what is normal for you
- Thoughts about suicide or dying
- New or worse depression
- Feeling agitated restless angry or irritable
- Other unusual changes in behavior mood
- Trouble sleeping

The truth is that if you take a drug for anxiety, you're twice as likely to be anxious and twice as likely to be depressed. But if that's not scary enough to cause patients to reconsider taking these pills, other side effects include:

- Loss of sexual ability

- Potential brain shrinkage

- Clinical worsening

- Heart disease risks

- Agitation

- Insomnia

- Lethargy

- Mental fog

- Emotional apathy

- Homicide

- Ten times more likely to get breast cancer

- Weight gain and obesity-related diseases like diabetes

These symptoms are the result of overstimulation or activation of the central nervous system. These meds are like hitting your head with a hammer causing drug induced brain injury. The removal of serotonin while trying to flood the brain with it creates chemical damage. It appears to work because you just injured it.

SSRI antidepressants block the removal of serotonin from the synapsis (important gaps) between neurons, in effect trying to flood these synapses with serotonin. Many studies confirm that the brain attempts to compensate for the impact of the SSRI's by reducing the brain's capacity to respond to serotonin. This leads to a loss of serotonin receptors that can reach 60%.

These toxic effects on the brain can lead to the emotional deterioration of patients. Prolonged SSRI antidepressant use can produce abnormal cell growth called neurogenesis. Some evidence suggests it decreases thalamic volumes (an important part of the brain) in children, which is connected to sensory systems, motor activity, emotion, memory, arousal and other sensorimotor association functions.

Bestselling author and psychiatrist, Peter R Breggin, M.D., warns prescribers of these drugs, therapists, patients and their families, "Antipsychotic drugs are highly toxic and produce many potentially severe and even lethal adverse effects such as chronic brain impairment CBI; atrophy of the brain; tardive dyskinesia [uncontrollable movements] including tardive psychosis [a delayed effect of the medication] and persistent cognitive impairment; neuroleptic malignant syndrome NMS [a life-threatening reaction to the drugs]; and metabolic syndrome including obesity elevated cholesterol, elevated blood sugar and potentially lethal diabetes."

Antipsychotic meds also cause drug-induced parkinsonism (DIP) in about 40% of patients. The percentage would be higher, but DIP resembles Parkinson's Disease (PD), causing patients to be misdiagnosed with PD.

Prescribing these pills ensures that doctors will have patients for life. They damage the frontal lobe and shrink the brain causing further pain and suffering for the patient. The longer these pills are taken, the more pills prescribed the more damage done.

## Do Antidepressants, Antipsychotic and Psychotropic Drugs Cure Symptoms?

Gwen Olsen, a former pharmaceutical sales rep and a victim of the drugs she once sold, explains that antipsychotic drugs don't fix brain abnormalities or balance brain chemicals. They suppress brain function retaining physical mobility and diminishing certain psychotic symptoms. These drugs grossly affect dopamine levels in the brain which is known to increase some people's vulnerability to psychosis.

Many studies have warned of the dangers and ineffectiveness of antidepressants:

- Men and women aged 24 to 30 years taking antidepressants found an increased rate of mortality, according to a recent Swedish study. When combined with other medications including antipsychotic drugs the rate continued to increase.

- According to a 2011 meta-analysis of 46 studies, the relapse rate for patients treated with antidepressants was 44.6%, while patients treated with placebos had a significantly lower rate of only 24.7%.

- A 2010 Minnesota evaluation of patient care within the state found that only 4.5% of more than 20,000 patients were in remission at 12 months. It seems the rest of the patients had become chronically afflicted with depression during and *probably as a result of their treatment.*

- A 2006 study of 1,255 suicides in Sweden (accounting for 95% of all suicides in the country) reported 32% of Scandinavian men and 52% of Scandinavian women filled a prescription for antidepressants in the 180 days prior to suicide.

- Juurlink, Mamdami, Kopp and Redelmier (2006) reviewed more than 1,000 cases of actual suicides in the elderly and found that during the first months of treatment, the SSRI antidepressants were associated with nearly a five-fold higher risk compared to other antidepressants.

Even the WHO has reported outcomes for psychiatric diagnosis to be much better in countries where these medications are not used or are used less frequently. So why does the Chemical Religion continue to deceive people into taking antipsychotic drugs like Zyprexa? The drug is linked to weight gain and causing diabetes—and made $4.7 billion in one year for the pharma company Eli Lilly (IMS Health 2005b). The company saw an opportunity and concealed the risk for diabetes until it produced a diabetes drug that they could market countering Zyprexa's effects. Big Pharma isn't in business to help you. They are in business to make money.

Even if someone *feels* that these psychoactive substances are helping them, they're not correcting an underlying chemical imbalance in their brain. They are potentially **creating neurological imbalances**. Most perceived improvements are the outward expression of damage of the frontal lobe.

## Maybe It's in Your Heart

We have patients who have lost children, others who have experienced devastating divorces, and others who have come from abusive relationships. Imagine if they came to us in their emotional distress or depression and we told them there must be something wrong with their brain. How offensive it is to be refused validation for emotional trauma! And yet this is how the Chemical Religion treats victims of heartache. Some doctors completely overlook the experiences causing their patients' depression and instead prescribe pills to numb their emotions. The antidepressants produce an altered mental state instead of helping patients through their pain on their journey to emotional healing.

Noel Hunter, PsyD, warns, "telling a person they are 'ill' for suffering or being sad serves to further alienate the individual. It often results in the person feeling defective and puts the problem inside the individual instead of recognizing that cultural and circumstantial factors are a problem. Studies have demonstrated over and over again that a biological illness perspective on human suffering leads to decreased empathy, increased desire for social distance and increased prejudice and discrimination."

If you had a tiger in your house, would you take a pill to decrease your anxiety about its presence? Would you then take another pill to sleep at night for fear the tiger would consume you? Or would you contact someone who knew something about tigers to help you deal with it and get it out of your life? The pill doesn't make anything go away. It doesn't fix broken relationships, emotional trauma or bring back what is lost.

Life is hard sometimes. Bad things happen and none of us can escape it all of the time. We've been conditioned to avoid pain rather than to face it, even though it's a human condition. When we avoid pain, it stays with us. We can't get past it. That's why we say that we're "going through something." We aren't meant to hold onto it, we're meant to allow it to go through us as we keep walking past it.

The hardships of life make us stronger, and more empathetic toward others. People who struggle with depression have to fight the temptation to isolate themselves, especially those whose emotions are numbed by prescription drugs. But we all need to find someone to walk with us. "Rejoice with those who rejoice; mourn with those who mourn" Romans 12:15 NIV. This is what relationship looks like.

Besides cultivating honest relationships with caring people, depression can also be addressed with counseling. A good counselor can help identify the root and give strategies to empower and overcome depression. They can lead us back to hope. A good counselor does not prescribe more meds.

Counselors might discuss setting goals and they can work with us to reach those goals. This creates hope! Hope creates the energy to set and reach more goals, which creates more hope! This is a never-ending cycle that, if followed, creates momentum in life. As this cycle goes on, self-confidence increases. Self-worth increases. The goal isn't the goals we're reaching towards. The goal is the person we become as we pursue each goal in life!

A good counselor will explain that the same part of the brain used to worry is the same part that you use to meditate. That means that worrying is meditating. Thinking and rehearsing all the things that could go wrong or that have gone wrong is meditating on the negative. However, we can think and hope and pray on the things that we would rather see in our future. We can ponder Bible scriptures, healthy perspectives and anything else for which we have to be thankful.

The Bible puts it this way in Philippians 4:8, "Whatever is true, whatever is noble, whatever is right, whatever is pure, whatever is lovely, whatever is admirable—if anything is excellent or praiseworthy—think about such things." (NIV)

It may seem impossible to meditate on affirmations or words of encouragement all day and it truly will take some refocusing for those who have allowed themselves to think negatively, but in her book *Switch on Your Brain*, Dr. Leaf has proven that the brain can change. With discipline anyone can learn to take thoughts captive and think on positive things and outcomes instead.

## Maybe It's in Your Spine

Sometimes people become depressed without having any idea why. They just don't feel like themselves anymore and it can't be traced back to some emotional trauma. Looking for hope they may go to a doctor who may tell them they have a chemical imbalance and give them a pill that will *cause* a chemical imbalance that wasn't there before. Or, if they've been reading this book, they might seek out a good chiropractor instead.

There's a whole field of study called biopsychology that seeks to understand how one's brain affects behavior. When the spine is misaligned, the nervous system is unable to properly send messages through the body. There are differences between nerve cells, but all of them respond to signals from other cells and conduct signals along their processes. Neurons in the brain are the chemical messengers that communicate with other cells. The role of a chiropractor is to maintain the balance in the central nervous system to make sure nerve cells are functioning correctly. Better spinal alignment means better communication and increased system efficiency. Better structure equals better function.

Your brain and behavior are directly linked. Spinal misalignment causes interference in the communication from your brain to the rest of your body. It can impact your thinking, your behavior, your ability to control your behavior, your mindset and more. That's why it's so important to your physical and emotional health to get regular adjustments.

The central nervous system governs how we perceive the world around us, how we learn from experience, how we remember, how we direct our movements and how we communicate with each other. This impacts our ability to live a healthy lifestyle and choose healthy behaviors. Drive-thru, pill-popping therapy ignores the root causes and comes with a whole new package of symptoms. Chiropractic care seeks out the source of symptoms and offers truly healing solutions.

## Maybe It's in Your Environment

Depression can sneak in when we are overextending ourselves, under stress at work or with family. We may feel overwhelmed. Thoughts of giving up begin to drown our drive to overcome. Environment can affect our overall mental health, but we are the only ones who have the power to help ourselves. Identifying what changes can be made to eliminate some of our stress comes with zero side-effects and can be truly empowering.

Asking ourselves some questions to identify the source and potential solutions is a good place to start in overcoming thoughts of helplessness. Am I in a toxic relationship that I know I need to escape? Do I need to set better boundaries with family or children? Is my job or commute too much? Maybe it's time to work on my resumé.

For some reason most of us avoid change. We're like the frog that's slowly being cooked even though we have the power to hop out anytime. Don't be the frog. Think about the steps you can take to have a happier life. Set goals. Don't give up on yourself. Think twice about getting on that drive-thru pill that will make you too lethargic and apathetic to take action.

## Maybe It's in Your Lifestyle

Most of us struggle to balance the things we *have* to do with the things we *want* to do, but we are thrown off when we try to also do the things *others* want us to do. This juggling act makes up the foundation of our lifestyle. It determines the way we eat when we're too busy to plan healthy meals. We start hitting the drive-thru and microwaving. An overly busy lifestyle also determines our sleep habits. We have to stay up late because there just aren't enough hours in the day. Even when we try to sleep, we're unable to rest. We lay in bed rehearsing all that's going on and wonder how it'll all work out.

Our busy schedules cause us stress. Our fast-food diet fills us with toxins. Our drive-thru healthcare fills us with more toxins. And our lack of sleep all contributes to our mental health.

Chronic stress damages the energy powerhouses of our body called mito-chondria. These energy factories produce ATP, the currency through which all cells and organs in our body do their work. Stress can be toxic to our body. It changes our body's chemistry and impacts our mental health and metabolism.

- Stress changes gene expression. The release of cortisol and adren-aline shut down certain non-essential systems in the body.
- Stress reduces the ability to metabolize and detoxify. It affects gut health and the ability to get toxins eliminated.

Changing our lifestyle sometimes means saying "NO." Of course, we won't have time to care for ourselves if we're always doing what everyone else wants us to do. We won't have time to exercise or get the 7-9 hours of sleep recommended for mental health if we don't practice setting better boundaries.

Exchanging a lifestyle that's ruled by external circumstances for a more proactive approach can alleviate a lot of stress. Live by intent instead. Living intentionally by setting goals the *S.M.A.R.T.* way will impact well-being. Goals should be:

**S**pecific

**M**easurable

**A**chievable

**R**ealistic

**T**imely

Overcoming stress and avoiding depression can often be achieved simply by changing the way we eat and by moving our body more.

The fastest way to change our mood is to exercise. (We talked about this in Chapter Five.) Increasing our oxygen intake alleviates stress. Exercise boosts the endorphins in the brain, which are neurotransmitters that promote pleasure. This helps manage day to day stress and boosts overall mood. We feel better about ourselves, more in control and are empowered to set new goals.

## How Does Exercise Make a Difference?

**Exercise pumps up your endorphins.** Physical activity helps bump up the production of your brain's feel-good neurotransmitters, called endorphins. Although this function is often referred to as a "runner's high," a rousing game of tennis or a nature hike can also contribute to this same feeling.

Have you ever gone for a run and came back feeling like you could do anything? This is due, in part, from that neurotransmitter in your brain.

**Exercise is meditation in motion.** After a fast-paced game of racquetball or several laps in the pool, you'll often find that you've forgotten the day's irritations and concentrated only on your body›s movements. As you begin to regularly shed your daily tensions through movement and physical activity, you may find that this focus on a single task, and the resulting energy and optimism, can help you remain calm and clear in everything you do. What's the result of feeling good and clearing your head? A good mood!

**Exercise improves your mood.** Regular exercise can increase self-confidence. It can relax you and it can lower the symptoms associated with mild depression and anxiety. Exercise can also improve your sleep, which is often disrupted by stress, depression and anxiety.

All these exercise benefits can ease stress levels and give us a sense of command. As for our mental health, it helps to reduce symptoms of stress, anxiety, depression and obsessive-compulsive disorder. Additionally, there's evidence that high-intensity training helps prevent the recurrence of anxiety and depression symptoms.

Exercise is so much more than fitting into your jeans or getting swimsuit ready. It's about showing value to yourself.

### Maybe It's in Your Gut

We talked about gut health in Chapter Two, but did you know that a major part of *mental* health starts in your gut? It's true: 85% - 95% of your serotonin is in your gut, which is why you may remember a time when you were nervous or sad and your belly was in knots.

When a significant disturbance occurs, our body responds with a rush of adrenaline and cortisol for what is often called the "fight or flight" reaction. We were designed with this God-given hormonal response so that we would be able to save our own lives in emergency situations. But the Chemical Religion has renamed what is more scientifically called acute stress response to acute stress *disorder* making it yet another opportunity to make money off our humanity.

Acute stress response shuts down our digestive system. Studies have shown that the activity of hundreds of genes responsible for enzymes that break down fats and detoxify prescription drugs, are negatively impacted by stress. Managing and limiting stress is important to gut health, as is adopting a healthy diet (as we discussed in Chapter Two). So, what's eating at you is as important as what you're eating.

Studies have shown that productive counseling, clearing the central nervous system and a healthy lifestyle including diet, exercise and gut health can make all the difference.

The Dream Center in Los Angeles co-founded by Pastor Matthew Barnett is a three-year program designed to get prostitutes, gang members and drug addicts off the streets. The program takes in hard cases and teaches them life skills, how to have a deep relationship with God and how to serve others. The success rate wasn't what they had hoped until they opened a clinic that offered spinal correction. They also began to focus more on health and fitness, changing the menu to offer an organic salad bar and high-quality supplements. The Dream Center taught their residents the importance of moving their bodies and offered exercise classes. They helped them to eliminate toxins and get physically healthy in every way. The stats of those who did *not* return to their old lifestyle improved by five times, making it one of the most successful rehabs in the U.S. It went from an 8% to a 40% success rate!

A similar study was done by several researchers who believed there was a correlation between mental disorders and endocrine deficiencies and blood sugar imbalances. Delinquent probationers were placed on restricted diets without processed food, sugar, caffeine and other additives. They also increased their consumption of fruits and vegetables. The results were impressive! The probationers' behavior and attitudes were significantly improved.

Orthomolecular psychiatry is the restoration of proper molecular balance of the brain. It's a dietary approach usually accompanied by vitamin and mineral supplementation and/or other therapies such as counseling. Orthomolecular psychiatry has been successful when tested on schizophrenic and bipolar patients who had been unresponsive to medication. They were fed diets containing the substances needed for proper brain function. If the brain doesn't have what it needs (and especially when it must also overcome drug toxicity) it will not function.

Unfortunately, we won't hear about this method for dealing with mental illness because it's inexpensive, uncomplicated and doesn't make money for the Chemical Religion.

Are you beginning to see a pattern here? Every ailment can be avoided or combatted with increased oxygen and exercise, healthy eating, avoiding toxins, spinal health and coming into a relationship with God.

They told my dad it was all in his head after his accident left him in pain and on meds, leaving us with no hope. The Chemical Religion doesn't cure anything with their pills. Their doctors are only taught medicine, not healing. We did what they told us to do and now my Daddy's gone, but that doesn't have to be anyone else's story.

Every patient I've worked with who refuses to believe there's hope prove themselves right, but everyone who receives hope and begins to believe they can be free can be saved. I want to be able to give people hope when they were told there is not hope. I want to provide another solution when they were given no other. I want to validate that it's not "all in your head." I want to care enough to stand with others and to find the cause that leads to their healing.

"Don't copy the behavior and customs of this world, but let God transform you into a new person by changing the way you think. Then you will learn to know God's will for you, which is good and pleasing and perfect" Romans 12:2 NLT.

**Hope is what gives hope.**

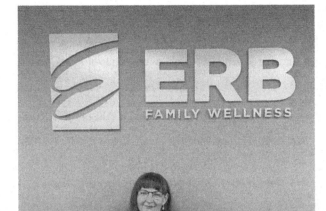

I was a physical education teacher and professional trainer for over 25 years. Moving to the U.S. and having to learn English was hard for me. For as long as I could remember, I had struggled with learning. I felt that I was capable of more, but there was a fog I didn't know how to overcome. Regardless, I kept working hard though I soon found myself working with clients to get them in better shape, while my own health was going slowly downhill. I refused to accept that it was aging causing my demise.

In 2009 I decided to have all my mercury fillings removed from my mouth. I began getting mercury fillings when I was seven years old. By the time I was 22 I had 16-18 silver fillings. That's when I noticed something was going really down south but I did not yet make the connection.

I noticed a growing inner anxiety after that. And the mental fog I had experienced as a child grew worse. I could not find a job after mine was downsized because I was incapable of reasoning or thinking clearly enough to make it through an interview successfully.

My symptoms continued to get worse. One night my husband and I were having a discussion that required us to brainstorm together. We got interrupted so we had to table it until the next day. When he brought it up, I had no recollection of the previous night's conversation. That's when we both realized something was wrong with me. We tried everything. No one could help me. I felt very lost.

I started having other symptoms including some that were menopausal. My emotions were so severe that I felt rage without cause. I had thoughts that scared me and at times had no care for the well-being of those around me or for myself. I was becoming an absolute nut case! I knew this wasn't me, but I was reacting with such strong outbursts that were controlling me.

The Lord led me to hope. I made a connection through our daughter's gymnastics to meet Dr. David. He noticed that my husband was limping. He invited Neal to come to his office for treatment. Neal and my daughter were checked, and my husband's limp was corrected.

When I first walked into the office of Erb Family Wellness, I could not read because I couldn't comprehend sentences longer than three words. I often felt lost in conversations.

Thanks to the doctors' knowledge about neurology and chiropractic understanding of how mercury affects the body, they recognized the problem and got to the cause. The mercury toxicity began when the first silver filling was placed in my mouth, and I grew more toxic as each additional one was added. Getting the mercury removed seems like a smart choice, but if precise protocol isn't followed, the poison is further released into your brain and body. That's why I got so sick after mine were removed.

Dr. Kimberly explained that I could be well if I detoxified my body. We started the process of removing heavy metals (chelating) and healing my gut. We continued this practice for the next ten years of my care. I regained every single function of my body and brain! I'm able to learn new and abstract things. I am also now capable of recalling pieces from my past that I had lost.

When I came to the office, I think my body was functioning like an 80–90-year-old woman. Ten years later at age 58 a full-body composition test proved I am functioning as a 43-year-old woman. My goal in the next 2-3 years is to function physically, mentally and emotionally as I was in my 30's and stay there for the rest of my life. I still refuse to believe that my age determines my health.

Thank you, Drs. David and Kimberly, for giving me my life back! – Dorota Konecky

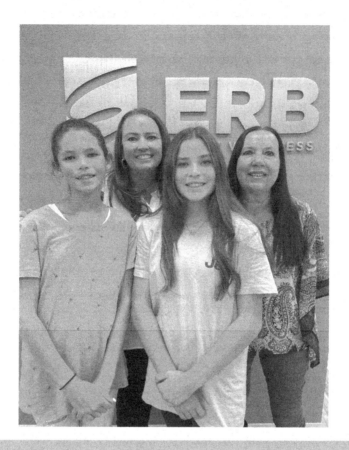

My husband, my daughter Candi and I started going to the Erbs in 2006. We are regulars. When we started, I had really bad allergies in the summer months. I have had these allergies since I was a child. We were also all taking anti-depressants. I was on other meds as well. We stopped all that pretty quickly after beginning our treatment at Erb Family Wellness. My allergies got better, and our overall emotional well-being improved significantly.

My daughter had two daughters, my beautiful grandchildren, while under the care of Erb Family Wellness. My granddaughters have had no vaccines, no medications, not so much as a Tylenol. They are 12 and 13 years old and have never had an earache. They have thrown up maybe three times in their lives. They are the healthiest kids ever!

We still get spinal adjustments once a week unless we are fighting off something. In that case we come more. My family hasn't needed to go to MDs and are drug free. Dr. David is so positive and uplifting. Sometimes encouragement is what we need most. He always prays for us and remembers from week to week what we have been going through and checks on us. - Renn Creasser

# CHAPTER 8
# GOD'S PROMISE: WHY ISN'T IT WORKING?

"Children are a gift from the LORD; they are a reward from him."

Psalm 127:3 NLT

One of our greatest joys has been seeing couples come in after they've tried everything to get pregnant. They have tried infertility meds like Clomid, in vitro fertilization (IVF), or even surrogate implantation. They've experienced the devastation of multiple miscarriages, and they are ready to give up. Patients like these have spent thousands of dollars on methods that have taken a toll on their emotions, their bodies and on their marriage. For these couples, making love has become something that adds additional pressure to their relationship rather than something that connects them. They walk in with just a mustard seed of hope, and we water it with action steps and support. We thank the Lord that so far, we have nearly a 100% success rate in helping our patients conceive. We're encouraged when patients come into our office to announce their pregnancies after making the changes we've prescribed.

Infertility has touched close to home, as I mourned with my cousin in her failed attempts to be a mom. Kelly struggled to get pregnant for years, until she had a back injury that led her to go see a chiropractor. She started getting adjusted and along came my sweet baby cousin! After the baby was born, Kelly stopped working on her spine and became infertile again—until she had another injury that sent her back to her chiropractor. Kelly's second baby is a confirmation that spinal health is a factor in fertility.

God has not only promised us children, but it's his command that we would multiply. I encourage my patients that he wouldn't give us a command that he hasn't equipped us to accomplish. His word says that he will withhold no good gift from us, and children are a gift and a reward.

### What Causes Infertility?

Infertility is like any of the other diseases we've talked about in previous chapters. We have to seek out the cause so we can heal our body. Some of the causes require lifestyle changes such as breaking free from addictions to alcohol, smoking and drugs, while others will require further digging to get to the source.

Women are usually the first to carry the burden of reproducing. Month after month they continue to be greeted by their period and wonder what's wrong with them. Some of the issues they face are listed below:

- Polycystic ovary syndrome (PCOS) is a hormonal disorder, a set of symptoms due to elevated androgens (male hormones) in females

- Endometriosis (a disease in which tissue that normally lines the inside of your uterus grows outside)

- Hormonal imbalances (your body is getting too little or too much of a specific hormone)

- Abortion (can affect potential for future pregnancies)

- Statins (reducing the body's ability to produce cholesterol, thus its ability to produce necessary hormones)

- Xenoestrogens (endocrine-disrupting chemicals like dioxins and pollutants)

- Subluxation

Usually after multiple failed attempts to conceive and months spent searching out answers in a woman's body, doctors will turn their attention to her partner. It surprises some that the male partner is either the sole or a contributing cause in about 40% of infertile couples.

- Testicular failure (the inability of the testicles to produce sperm and the male hormone testosterone)

- Eculatory disorder (premature, retarded or retrograde ejaculation). Premature ejaculation occurs before or very soon after penetration. Retarded ejaculation happens when ejaculation is slow to occur. Retrograde ejaculation occurs when, at orgasm, the ejaculate is forced back into the bladder rather than through the urethra and out the end of the penis.

- Sperm issues (low or absent sperm count, problems with sperm shape, movement, delivery)

- Varicoceles (an enlarged vein in the scrotum and testicle, usually found on the left side)

- Cell phone radiation (EMFs diminish sperm count and can cause sperm damage)

- Statins (reducing the body's ability to produce cholesterol, thus its ability to produce necessary hormones)

- Xenoestrogens (endocrine-disrupting chemicals like dioxins and pollutants that affect sperm)

- Prostate biopsy (can damage the prostate causing inability of erection)

- Prostate removal (majority of men never achieve erection again)

- Heavy metals (accumulate in testicles from shots and silver fillings)

- Blood pressure meds (effect ability for erection)

- Subluxation

- Lifestyle factors, such as obesity or smoking

Surprisingly, our fertility comes under attack before we're even born! A landmark study found 93% of blood samples taken from pregnant women and 80% from umbilical cords tested positive for traces of the genetically modified chemicals that would have to have come from eating GM crops and consuming meat, milk and eggs from farm livestock fed GM corn.

We've already established the risks associated with chemicals in pesticides like Roundup and GMOs in Chapter Two, but reproductive issues like PCOS are another reason to do everything in our power to limit our vulnerability to it. Several studies have identified Roundup or its components as disruptors of hormone function such as estrogen and progesterone necessary to reproducing. Roundup can contribute to our hormonal problems and cause PCOS. It may even cause birth abnormalities.

Billions of dollars have been awarded to people whose lives have been tragically impacted by the harmful effects of this pesticide, even if the FDA is still calling it safe. And now there's evidence that reveals these and other toxins can be passed to our unborn babies!

It should seem suspicious that most of the research used to prove the safety of GM crops has been funded by the industry itself, but when unbiased studies are performed, a different story is told. Traces of Bt toxin found in pesticides and genetically modified crops were discovered in the blood of 28 out of 30 pregnant moms and in the umbilical cords of 24 out of 30 of their babies. A nonpregnant group was also tested, and traces of the poisonous chemical were found in the blood of 27 out of the 39 women tested.

## Could the Chemicals Found in the Blood of Nonpregnant Women Effect Their Future Children and Grandchildren?

Chemicals and meds are finding their way into infants before they've even emerged from our wombs, but maybe parents aren't the only ones transferring the effects.

The history of the drug Diethylstilbestrol's (DES) use is quite extensive. It was first used to *prevent* miscarriages in pregnant women but is used today as an emergency contraceptive in the event a woman has unprotected sex. It's also used "when your birth control doesn't work correctly" implying that it can be used to *cause an abortion.*

We're still trying to wrap our brains around the evolution of this pill, given to women from 1930 to 1971 (when the FDA banned its use in pregnant women) with the intentions of preventing miscarriage that's now used for aborting unwanted babies and preventing pregnancy. Through the years DES has been prescribed for a long list of other reasons and ailments.

- To treat breast cancer
- Postpartum lactation suppression
- Menopausal symptoms
- To treat lack of estrogen issues like infertility and some cancers
- Gonorrheal vaginitis
- To treat excessive height in girls
- Prostate cancer
- Atrophic vaginitis

Despite the warnings from the DES developer biochemist Sir Charles Edward Dodds of its potentially cancerous effects if used as a regular contraceptive pill, pharmaceutical companies still recommend that doctors prescribe it. It turns out the drug's effects have been found to be harmful for at least three generations from pregnant mother to her children's children for its ability to cross the placenta and enter the fetal bloodstream where it accumulates in the baby's reproductive tract. Daughters and granddaughters have suffered:

- Vaginal cancer
- Breast cancer
- Miscarriages
- Clear cell adenocarcinoma of the vagina

- Premature births
- Ectopic pregnancies
- Earlier menopause

There have been many lawsuits against a group of DES manufacturers alleging that their mothers' ingestion of DES caused injuries, including the 1980's *Sindell v. Abbott Laboratories*, a California Supreme Court case that drew attention to the longsuffering in family lines, occurring from the use of the drug in pregnant women.

In *Sindell v. Abbott Laboratories* two DES daughters, Judith Sindell and Maureen Rogers won their case against the drug manufacturers when the court established the precedent of market share liability. Because the effects aren't always seen until children become adults, it is difficult to hold a specific pharmaceutical company accountable. In the shared liability, the entire market is responsible for a share of a settlement when the individual manufacturer cannot be identified.

When DES was being developed as a powder, men in the lab developed breasts from inhalation. Sons exposed to the drug in the womb and grandsons have suffered:

- A penis under two inches in length
- Epididymal cysts

- The absence of one or both testes
- Testicular cancer

- Underdevelopment of
  the testes

DES increases risk of cardiovascular disease and diabetes in prenatally exposed women. Mothers administered DES during pregnancy have an increased risk for breast cancer and mortality. Even the FDA has listed the drug as a known carcinogen.

Diethylstilbestrol isn't the only toxic substance being inherited by grandchildren.

Michael Skinner of Washington State University is a pioneer in epigenetics, the study of inherited changes in gene expression. He's the senior author of a study published in the journal *PLoS One*. Skinner's research group found that pregnant rats exposed to high doses of dioxin (and other chemicals) passed down the negative health effects to their *great* granddaughters. The young rats had nearly eight times higher rates of developing cysts and other ovarian problems during puberty, even though they were not directly exposed compared to the control rats. Third generation rats also showed an increase in ovarian disease.

Skinner reported:

- 47% of third generation females had early puberty.

- First-generation offspring had more prostate disease and two types of ovarian disease.

- Kidney disease, changes in puberty and ovarian disease were more prevalent in the great grandkids.

- Sperm in third generation males showed modifications in gene expression in 50 regions of DNA as a result of their ancestors' dioxin exposure.

Another study performed on mice found:

- A decline in fertility in the third generation following dioxin exposure to pregnant mice.

- Increased incidence of premature birth in mice exposed in utero, as well as in three subsequent generations.

The last thing our grandparents and great grandparents wanted to pass down to us is infertility, and we would never want that to be the legacy we leave for our own children and grandchildren. It's not too late to clean out the junk heirlooms and start building a healthy inheritance for our future offspring. Avoid EDCs, xenoestrogens and polysorbate 80. They're fertility sabotagers!

The National Institute of Environmental Health Sciences defines endocrine-disrupting chemicals (EDCs) as "chemicals that interfere with the body's endocrine system and produce adverse developmental, reproductive, neurological and immune effects." It's comprised of glands that are distributed throughout the body some of which are the hypothalamus, pituitary, thyroid and reproductive organs. EDCs can be in the air, food, water, skincare products and other household items. They affect our health in many ways including our ability to reproduce. They can cause:

- Metabolic issues
- Abnormalities in sex organs
- Endometriosis
- Early puberty
- Altered nervous system function
- Immune function
- Neurological and learning disabilities.

- Respiratory problems
- Alterations in sperm quality and fertility
- Diabetes
- Obesity
- Cardiovascular problems
- Certain cancers

When unborn babies and children are exposed, developmental abnormalities and an increased risk for a variety of diseases later in life have been linked to EDCs. Extreme caution should be used when pregnant or breastfeeding, as they've been found to cross the placenta and become concentrated in the fetus' circulation. Some EDCs can also be transferred from mother to infant through breast milk.

Xenoestrogens are another concern plaguing humanity and diminishing our ability to reproduce. Whether natural or man-made, xenoestrogens such as those in pharmaceuticals, plasticizers, polychlorinated biphenyls (PCBs), organochlorines, polyfluoroalkyls (PFOAs), phthalates and pesticides are seen by the body as an overload of estrogens causing tumors and cysts, including PCOS and uterine fibroids.

If you're suffering from any of these symptoms, you might have estrogen dominance:

- Irritability
- Anxiety
- Hot flashes
- Insomnia
- Weight gain
- Migraines
- Depression

Dioxins are xenoestrogens described by *The Medical News Today* as, "a group of highly toxic chemical compounds that are harmful to health. They can cause problems with reproduction, development and the immune system. They can also disrupt hormones and lead to cancer." They come from natural sources such as volcanoes but also through other burning processes such as commercial, waste incineration and burning with many fuels. Chlorine bleaching is another way we are exposed to dioxins.

They're impossible to completely avoid, but every precaution should be considered since it can take between seven and eleven years for dioxin's radioactivity to fall to half its original level within the body.

## Here Are the Top 10 Sources to Avoid

1. Commercially raised meat and dairy products

2. Anything that contains insecticide or pesticide residues

3. Tap water

4. Paraben

5. Phthalates (soft plastics for packaging)

6. Artificial food additives

7. Foods that contain soy protein and soy protein isolate

8. Dryer sheets

9. Birth control pills and conventional hormone replacement therapy (HRT)

10. Disposable menstrual products (look for organic, non-GMO)

It seems that the market for things to make people sick, infertile and dead are among the highest in demand. We're constantly reading labels and doing research to be the gatekeepers of our home and for our patients. Sometimes we just look at each other and ask, "Why?" Why would companies even consider exposing people to such atrocities?

Polysorbate 80 is one of those ingredients that caused our heads to shake in disgust. Polysorbate 80 is used in the pharmaceutical and cosmetic industry. It can be found in vitamins, lotions, medical preparations like vitamin oils, vaccines and intravenous preparations listed under the alias's Tween 80, canarcel and alkest. It's used as an excipient in tablets and in vaccines. It's an emulsifier to enhance the chemicals to the blood in the brain. Polysorbate 80 may even make way for other vaccines to cross the blood-brain barrier allowing the metals to build up on the brain. By the way, it's also an emulsifier in soft serve ice cream. It's smooth and creamy poison!

**The Material Safety Data Sheet for polysorbate 80 says:**

- Slightly flammable to flammable in presence of heat
- Slightly hazardous in case of skin contact (irritant), of eye contact (irritant), of ingestion, of inhalation
- May cause adverse reproductive effects based on animal test data, no human data found
- May cause cancer based on animal test data, no human data found
- May affect genetic material

Whenever you see the phrase "no human data found," it doesn't mean a product is safe for consumption. At best it means they don't *know* if it's harmful. Often times it means concerns have been raised but, "let's just see how far we can take this until the item gets pulled off the market." In the case of polysorbate 80, there has been animal testing that proves the potential it could cause similar issues in humans. If there is even a potential that something could cause us to get cancer, we're out! Why does the Chemical Religion insist on taking chances with lives? Nevertheless, GMO products will continue to be sold while research accumulates to discredit it. Unsuspecting consumers will be the guinea pigs for studies on the effects of polysorbate 80 on humans.

An article based on a Slovakian study published in the journal Food and Chemical Toxicology in 1993 by Joseph Mercola, DO suggests polysorbate 80 might cause infertility. Baby female rats were injected with polysorbate 80 at days 4-7 after birth. Many fertility issues occurred including accelerated maturation, changes to their vagina and womb lining, hormonal changes, ovary deformities and degenerative follicles. The relative weight of the uterus and ovaries were decreased, and the rats' ovaries were also damaged and no corpora lutea (a mass of progesterone-secreting endocrine tissue that forms immediately after ovulation). Such severe deformities to the ovary can lead to infertility. It literally dries up the womb.

Besides ridding ourselves from these things, we can take further measures to heal our bodies from the effects of xenoestrogens, EDCs and polysorbate 80. Supplements, clean diet, detox and spinal adjustments to boost our natural immune response are the hope that we'll offer in our final chapter.

## Miscarriage: Why Joy Turns to Sorrow

We have too many dear friends and patients who've suffered the devastation of miscarriage. The numbers can be discouraging with research that estimates between 10% and 20%, or as many as one in four known pregnancies end in miscarriage. Evolutionary geneticist William Richard Rice of the University of California, Santa Barbara goes so far as to say half of all successful fertilizations end in miscarriage. What is causing our unborn babies to die in our womb?

Professor Don M. Huber of Purdue University has discovered a completely new, unknown organism within genetically modified crops that can cause miscarriages in farm animals. We're finding that unborn humans are dying from exposure, too. Even the American Medical Association suggests that pesticide residues in food may account for a large proportion of the roughly 100,000 unsuccessful pregnancy attempts in fertility clinics across North America.

The evidence against GM's ambush on fertility continues to build. Dr. Medardo Avila-Vazquez led a study of people living in Monte Maíz, an Argentine town in the heart of a GM soy and corn growing area. He's a physician who has spearheaded investigations into the health of populations exposed to glyphosate herbicide spraying on GM glyphosate-tolerant soy and corn. The doctor found that the women in Monte Maíz suffer miscarriages at three times the national average and babies are born with birth defects at twice the national average!

The study also found:

- A higher environmental exposure to glyphosate had an increased frequency of reproductive disorders such as miscarriage and birth defects.

- Women who consumed the most pesticides reduced their chance of having a live birth by 26% compared to woman who consumed the least amount of pesticides.

- Women who consumed the least pesticides reduced their risk of miscarriage to 7%, compared to the 34% chance of miscarriage by women consuming the most pesticides.

A study by *JAMA* calculated that if women replaced just one serving per day of high pesticide residue produce with one serving per day of low pesticide residue produce, their chances of a live birth would improve by 88%. All of these studies are offering the same encouragement that we give. Change your diet; change your possibilities.

## What Part Do Vaccines Play in Miscarriage?

In Chapter One we shocked you with the truth that several vaccines are made from human fetuses. The market for fetuses continues to grow with vaccine use, but it can now be found in a growing number of cosmetic companies and food companies. Ever wondered what "artificial flavors" mean? Often times it's code for flavor receptors engineered from *human embryonic kidney cells* (HEK 293, fetal cell line popular in pharmaceutical research). These artificial taste buds can tell product developers which products the public will crave. Repulsive!

While many couples are trying to have babies, others are aborting their babies, which unbeknownst to them, will be sold. Nor do the women applying the child's remains to their skin have any idea how their products were developed. It's known as Processed Skin Proteins (PSP), developed at the University of Lausanne to heal burns and wounds by regenerating traumatized skin.

There doesn't seem to be any risk factors for the living in using products associated with unborn babies, but for some pregnant, vaccinated women the injection creates an immune response within their body that now recognizes fetal tissue within the womb as something to attack. The vaccine containing the fetus taught the body to see an unborn baby as a virus and causes a miscarriage.

## The Assault on Our Youth's Fertility

Pharmaceutical companies have been pushing fear upon moms to get their preteen daughters a vaccine they say will protect them from certain sexually transmitted diseases. The human papillomavirus (HPV) vaccine can be given to kids as early as age nine. Officially, the CDC recommends that boys and girls ages 11 or 12 get it. Our daughter was still playing dress up with her dolls at that age! I assure you that with proper supervision and parenting, it's highly unlikely your kids will be having sex so young. But just in case, what are the risks, and do they outweigh the risks of the vaccine itself?

Wikipedia says, "About 90% of HPV infections cause no symptoms and resolve spontaneously within two years." But there's still that 10% chance that sexually active children who are not routinely checking on the health of their sexual organs (including their anus and mouth) could become infected. If an HPV infection persists it could possibly result in either warts or precancerous lesions. These lesions increase the risk of cancer of the cervix, vulva, vagina, penis, anus, mouth or throat depending on their location. But does that 10% chance that an issue in your sexually active teen will be overlooked (along with the chance that your teen will actually become sexually active) justify the risks associated with the vaccine?

The HPV vaccine wasn't introduced to Australians until 2007. Like many other vaccines taking credit for decreasing numbers, prior to this vaccine introduction, the incidence and mortality rate of cervical cancer was already steadily declining. According to a study, the rates for 20 to 69-year old's in Australia were more than halved in the decade prior to 2000, which was long before the vaccine made its debut. But upon the introduction of the vaccine, other attacks on women's health and fertility loomed.

In a series of cases featuring three girls in different parts of Australia, the first case had her first period at age 13 in 2007. In 2008 she had three rounds of the HPV vaccine. By the time she was 16 years old, she developed irregular menses, gradually progressing to infrequent menstrual periods (oligomenorrhea), then to an abnormal absence of menstruation (amenorrhea). Finally, in 2011 she was diagnosed with premature ovarian failure (POF). Her doctor put her on an oral contraceptive, even though she was not sexually active. This, by the way, did nothing to heal her body from the damage inflicted upon her reproductive system.

Further bad news for the poor girl came when she was advised of her newly acquired need for bone strength preservation. POF is one of the greatest risk factors for osteoporosis. Lowered bone mineral density begins with diminished ovarian function and inferior bone density in teens is a factor in the development of osteoporosis. Take a pill, take a shot, and you may be a patient for life.

The 20-year-old girl in the case series was given her first HPV4 at 12 years old, the second vaccination about three months later and the third vaccination at about age 13 and a half. A gynecologist recorded, "although her periods were reasonably normal, she was put on the pill the next year because coping with her periods made her anxiety and depression symptoms worse." By the time the girl was 18, her pathologist said her ovarian appearance was "consistent with that of a woman in her late forties" and described the macroscopic appearance of the girl's ovary as "cystic and disrupted." This girl was also advised of her impending bone density issues.

The last patient emphasized, "prior to this [HPV vaccination], my periods were like clockwork." The period due after the third vaccination dose was two weeks late. It was the first late period she had ever experienced. The next period occurred two months later. Her next and final menstruation occurred nine months later, which happened to be approximately one year after completion of the third HPV4 vaccination.

The three girls all developed premature ovarian insufficiency, along with other issues before they were even sexually active.

Australian reviews of this vaccine's safety research have been criticized even by top vaccine experts for not having the follow through necessary to justify promotion to the public. Younger person safety studies lacked full control group and had very small numbers of young females receiving all three vaccinations. One of the two studies had lost more than half to 12-month follow-up even though these 10 to 15-year-olds were to be followed for one year after their first vaccination for safety. Only 40.4% of boys studied (205 in total) completed 12-month safety follow-up in this designated safety study. One 15-year-old boy died suddenly 27 days after his second vaccination. I wonder if they didn't complete the study because they weren't liking the results.

### Has the Pill Become the Cure-All for Typical Teen Traumas?

Teens are moody, they get acne and they're often overwhelmed by their menstrual cycles. We don't want to belittle them for what they go through, especially for those who have out of the normal struggles with their puberty experiences. But it's important not to get caught up in fixing something that's natural with something that's unnatural.

Our daughter was late in comparison to her peers to start her period. Zoey had not been exposed to all of the hormone disrupting, accelerating maturation chemicals we've now brought to the light in this chapter. Young ladies are developing and becoming women as early as fourth grade these days. Our daughter experienced these changes naturally, without the forced push from all the poisonous crap.

Unfortunately, young girls lack the maturity to manage all the hormonal changes. Many suffer from heightened symptoms or irregular cycles because of their diet and exposure to all the toxins. I'm sure you can guess that your OBGYN has a pill for that, too. And so it begins: the Chemical Religion inserting itself into our youths' reproductive process.

It's unbelievable to me how many of our daughter's friends were on birth control at such young ages for reasons completely unrelated to potential pregnancy. Menstruation is a normal part of God's design for fertility. Interfering with the Creator's design is disrupting the fertility process. When considering irregular cycles, cysts, cramps, or whatever the issues our daughters might be facing, remember to look for the cause rather than for a pill, which opens the door for some more serious health risks.

Combination contraception, known simply as "the pill" may or may not regulate periods, will probably prevent unwanted pregnancy and will increase a young woman's risk for all kinds of other unwanted issues.

- Breast cancer
- Depression
- Weight gain
- Stroke
- Cervical cancer
- VTE (blood clots in the veins that can cause disability or death)
- Heart arrhythmias
- Electrolyte imbalance
- Gallbladder problems
- Embolisms
- Sudden death

Taking the pill increases the risk of stroke. It destroys one of the layers within the blood vessels called the tunica intima, creating a weakness and ruining the blood vessel's ability to pump blood. The risk of ischemic stroke is higher for those on the pill, especially for those who also have a history of migraines. One study was performed over the course of ten years on 10,000 women between the ages of 25 to 29. Women this age only have a 2.7x risk of ischemic stroke, but the risk nearly doubles to 4x if she uses oral contraceptives. It increases even more significantly to 23x if she uses oral contraceptives and has migraines with aura.

Breast cancer risk is another disease to consider when deciding to take the pill or give it to your daughter. A recent Danish cohort study reported a 20% increased risk of breast cancer among current and recent hormonal contraceptive users.

Taking the pill can cause VTE (blood clots in the veins that can cause disability or death). Observational studies found one to three additional cases of VTE among 10,000 women taking combination contraceptives for one year. These blood clots in the veins can cause serious injury or death.

Hormonal contraception has also been associated with subsequent use of antidepressants and a first diagnosis of depression, especially among adolescents. First your daughter is put on the pill, then she's put on an antidepressant, then she's put on a diabetes drug. And the pills will just keep coming.

Cervical cancer risk increases after five years of taking birth control pills. Young girls are starting so early and will likely be on oral contraceptives for years and years to come without realizing the dangers.

Bayer has resolved more than 19,000 lawsuits so far over one popular birth control pill, Yaz/Yasmin. The lawsuits allege the pills caused blood clots, gallbladder problems, heart attacks and strokes. Many believe that Bayer intentionally concealed knowledge of risks and misled the public about supposed benefits of the medications which isn't hard to believe given the company's history.

Bayer's roots are connected to WWII, with its parent company having close ties to the Third Reich. There are records suggesting it paid Nazi officials for access to prisoners for human experimentation. Bayer also promoted a cold and cough medicine for children containing heroin until 1912. And let's not forget that they also bought the deadly pesticide Roundup from Monsanto containing glyphosate. But they really care about people, right?

Maggie Yunker suffered a life-altering stroke at age 20 after switching to Yaz, Bayer's birth control pill. Her doctor recommended it to clear up her acne and relieve period symptoms. The trusting girl began taking the new birth control pill and later developed multiple blood clots that broke free and traveled to her brain. Once in the brain, the clots cut off blood flow and caused a stroke. Bayer settled Maggie's claim for $237,000. She told the Chicago Tribune, "I didn't think anything bad could happen, especially since a doctor was giving it to me . . . Any medicine has risk factors, but when you're 20 you don't think about it."

Unfortunately, people of all ages have trusted in the Chemical Religion, overlooking warning labels until they're faced with the reality that it *can* happen to them. Roughly 20,000 women were injured or died after taking Yaz, resulting in lawsuits similar to Maggie Yunker's. And that's just one contraceptive's story.

When birth control isn't working to cure a girl's acne, she may be prescribed Accutane. Teen girls and boys are highly cautioned even by M.D.s when taking this dangerous pill (see Chapter Ten for more on Accutane). They're required to have blood work done every month to ensure it hasn't begun to affect their liver and that females haven't become pregnant. It's imperative that this drug not be taken when pregnant or nursing, as Accutane dries every gland in your body putting youth and adults at risk for future infertility problems and side effects such as:

- Miscarriage

- Congenital disabilities

- Premature labor

- Death in babies

If there's one thing we're trying to get readers to understand, it's that just because the FDA allows a product or drug to hit the market and just because the pharmaceutical company has a heartwarming commercial that promises you can get your life back and just because your medical doctor prescribes a medication, it does not mean the products and drugs are safe. It does not mean that they have been thoroughly tested.

## Are Artificial Fertility Methods the Cure for the Infertility Effects of Prescription Drugs and Chemicals?

Deciding to write the next part of this chapter is something we didn't take lightly. The ability to reproduce and the desire to do so were innately created in us from the beginning of time. The desperate cries of those longing to have children are some of the most moving we've experienced as D.C.s. Fertility can be a sensitive discussion and the last thing we want to do is make someone feel judged for the choices they've made or for the one's they might still be considering. Please understand that our hearts are to present the truth, which isn't being shared. We want to expose the lies that are costing people their health and their future. We hope to accomplish this without bringing shame to anyone.

Clomid is usually the first step in the infertility journey for couples. Healthline.com describes it as "an oral medication that is often used to treat certain types of female infertility. The drug works by making the body think that your estrogen levels are lower than they are, which causes the pituitary gland to increase secretion of follicle stimulating hormone, or FSH, and luteinizing hormone, or LH." Simply put, it stimulates the brain to produce more eggs.

As you may have guessed, this drug comes with some significant side effects as well. A few of those reactions are listed plainly, the ones that don't seem so bad when one is hopeful for the possibility of being able to have a baby. Those effects listed below are what has been documented from studies *premarketing* or *before* the drug has been marketed.

- Hot flashes

- Mood swings

- Breast discomfort or tenderness

- Nausea or vomiting

- Bloating

- Headaches

Other side effects include:

- Heavier menses or irregular menstrual bleeding

- Dizziness or lightheadedness

- Trouble sleeping

If you don't believe patients are guinea pigs, then you don't understand *postmarketing* reporting. Wikipedia defines it as, "The practice of monitoring the safety of a pharmaceutical drug or medical device *after* it has been released on the market and is an important part of the science of pharmacovigilance." Think about that for a moment. Drugs are recommended by doctors who will use their patients' experience as further research into the safety or risks of the product. Would you want to take a medication without fully knowing the risks? Do you want to be the one to discover another adverse reaction from something that you're told will make you feel better? With your help, your M.D. will report on the side effects you experience. These, often more severe side effects, are more difficult to find, and are often the ones that would cause one to weigh out the risks versus the benefits more thoughtfully. Here are some of the postmarketing reports of Clomid:

- Arrhythmia (abnormal heart rate or rhythm), chest pain, hypertension, palpitation, tachycardia (fast heart rate), thrombophlebitis.

- All kinds of eye issues such as cataract, eye pain, macular edema (swelling throughout your body), optic neuritis (inflammation of the optic nerve leads to vision loss), photopsia (eye floaters), retinal hemorrhage (bleeding from the blood vessels in the retina), retinal thrombosis (blood clot blocks the vein, temporary or prolonged loss of vision).

- Hepatic hemangiosarcoma (tumor in the liver), hepatocellular carcinoma (liver cancer), fibrocystic disease, breast carcinoma (cancer), endometrial cancer, astrocytoma (brain tumor), pituitary tumor, neurofibromatosis (nervous system disease that causes skin defects and tumors on nerve tissues), glioblastoma multiforme (the most aggressive brain cancer), brain abscess.

- Ovary issues such as; luteoma (a tumor occurring during pregnancy), dermoid cyst of the ovary, ovarian carcinoma (cancer), hydatiform mole (clusters formed in uterus around a dying unborn baby), choriocarcinoma (a fast growing cancer that grows in the womb), melanoma, myeloma, renal cell carcinoma (cancer that begins in the kidney or ureters), Hodgkin's lymphoma (cancer of the immune system), tongue carcinoma (cancer), bladder carcinoma (cancer), migraines, seizure, stroke, fainting, pancreatitis, endometriosis, ovarian hemorrhage, tubal Pregnancy, uterine hemorrhage, reduced endometrial thickness.

- Rapid weight gain.

- Psychological and emotional side effects.

Clearly, a woman is risking quite a bit of her own health (and even her life) in hopes this pill will enable her to conceive. How devastating it would be to get pregnant only to birth a baby with serious health diseases? Many women suffered such a fate for the following postmarketing reports fetal and neonatal to be made known.

- Cleft lip/palate, imperforate anus, tracheoesophageal fistula, diaphragmatic hernia, omphalocele

- Abnormal bone development, skeletal malformations of skull/face/nasal passages/jaw/hand limb/foot/spine/joints Neural tube defect, anencephaly, meningomyelocele), microcephaly, hydrocephalus

- Septal heart defect, muscular ventricular septal defect, patent ductus arteriosus, tetralogy of fallot, coarctation of aorta and Hypospadias, cloacal exstrophy

- Eye malformed, lens malformed/cataract

- Neuroectodermal tumor, thyroid tumor, hepatoblastoma, lymphocytic leukemia

PubMed.gov states, "Alarming data has emerged from animal studies, although controversial results come from human studies. There is some evidence regarding a possible association of CC [clomiphene citrate] exposure and fetal malformations, mainly neural tube defects and hypospadias, which would require further investigation to allow safer use of this useful drug." Those studies will likely come from patients and lawsuits against the drug for its effects.

Now, imagine going into the doctor with fertility issues and coming out with a prescription for diabetes that you don't have. Metformin is usually prescribed for diabetes, but it's sometimes given to women with PCOS because it can also stimulate ovulation. I think I'd have to wonder how such a drug could also be affecting my glucose levels, but I guess if it works then it's worth it? I'll give you the facts and let you decide.

The Cochrane Library's systematic review of the drug's effects on fertility concluded, "While metformin alone might increase the odds of ovulation in some people, studies have *not* found that it increases pregnancy rates or live birth rates." So, women are taking a pill that is now being sued for having distributed several batches with as much as 16.5 times the limit of NDMA, a carcinogen that causes many forms of cancer including ovarian and testicular.

When a couple has tried everything else and still has not been able to reproduce, invitro fertilization (IVF) becomes an option for those who can afford it. On average, an IVF cycle costs $12,000 plus medications, which typically run another $3,000 to $5,000. There's only about a 40% success rate (at best) for a process that runs about $20,000 **for each attempt**. In other words, if at first you don't succeed, the M.D.s welcome you to invest another $20,000 for another chance. We've had patients come to us after running out of resources feeling hopeless and taken advantage of in their desperation to grow their family. But even with all the money spent, the risks associated with IVF were not made clear.

The dismal 40% chance of pregnancy comes with health risks for mom and baby. PubMed.gov concluded a study that showed an 80% increased risk of cerebral palsy in the IVF group and another study that showed IVF-ET and current IUD use play dominant roles in the occurrence of ectopic pregnancy.

Whether from ectopic pregnancy or miscarriage, losing a baby is the kind of pain that sits on your chest so heavy you feel like you can't breathe. It makes you wonder if it's even worth trying to catch your next breath.

We remember our excitement when I took a pregnancy test on the flight from Zimbabwe back to the U.S. The whole plane celebrated with us as an announcement was made. But our joy was short lived and would soon be replaced with a deep emptiness. With each drop of blood, as I lay still with my legs pressed together tightly, a new dream would be mourned. The dream of seeing my baby for the first time, the dream of the first steps and what our baby would have grown up to be; it was sorrow against hope, and sorrow won.

The pain we experienced losing our baby has fueled our passion to see our patients conceive and deliver healthy babies. We don't want anyone to go through such loss, though many of our new patients come to us afraid to try again. We've been honored to offer hope and healing to couples as their heart grieves the babies they've lost.

Genesis 1:28a (CEV) says, "God gave them his blessing and said: Have a lot of children!" We cannot keep putting our hope in the Chemical Religion when they're shoving pills down our throats and forcing vaccines on us that can potentially rob us of our God-given reward and promise.

God doesn't want us to carry shame and regret for what we didn't know. He's a loving God; He's a good God, and He has made a way for us to overcome and to be fruitful. We promise to show you how you can align yourself with his design for your body to heal itself and overcome the effects of the Chemical Religion. Our past is covered by the cross and our future is full of hope. Keep reading!

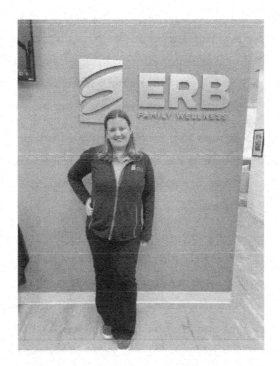

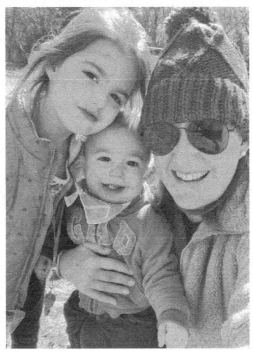

I started working at Erb Family Wellness in 2014. A week after I started, the metabolic testing was launched in their office. Metabolic is an advanced test that uses blood and urine to determine many risk factors such as cancer. It can tell you what your body is missing and can even give indicators of the kinds of toxins you are being exposed to.

My gynecologist told me I had a uterine fibroid the size of my fist. She warned me that it would make getting pregnant and carrying a baby to full term very difficult. She said that if I wanted kids, I needed to get pregnant as soon as possible.

I took the advice of the doctors I now worked for and began getting chiropractic adjustments from them. I also did my first round of metabolic testing and had great results as I followed the plan it customized for me. When I took the test again it showed how hard I had been working. I followed the updated plan, but I wasn't thinking when I had my house sprayed for bugs. This time when I was retested my markers were poor from the toxic chemicals. I stayed strong on the plan, and I did the testing again. Finally, I was all cleared, and BOOM! A month later I was pregnant with my first baby at 36 years old.

My husband and I were so surprised, as was my OBGYN! She warned me that it was a high-risk pregnancy, so I gave my body exactly what it needed based on metabolic. I put all my faith in Dr. Kimberly Erb to get my baby and I through the pregnancy. She continued to adjust my spine and encouraged me in the practices of toxicity elimination, having a positive mindset, proper nutrition and exercise. I didn't even fill my prenatal prescription because I knew I was getting everything I needed from the supplements recommended by the personalized plan that I was on.

Pregnancy hormones cause fibroids to grow. Mine had grown to be the size of my baby by the end of my pregnancy. This put us further at risk making a C- section our only delivery option. This might have been disappointing except that a couple days before my daughter was born my doctor confessed that she didn't expect I could carry to term. I believe 100%, with all my heart, that God led me to the Erbs and that supplements and chiropractic care are what got me through the high-risk pregnancy.

After my C-section which was a "classic cut" meaning all future pregnancies will have to be delivered C-section, I did hyperbaric. Dr. Kimberly recommended hyperbaric oxygen therapy because it would speed up the healing process in my incision. My OBGYN was astonished that after only seven days my scar had healed so quickly it looked like it had been several months!

My husband and I wanted to try again for another baby. I decided to have surgery to remove the fibroid before trying. It was a rough road at first. We suffered a few early miscarriages and had to have a D&C with the last one. In all, I had three surgeries before getting pregnant with Jacob. The C-section, the fibroid removal and the D&C, but after the last surgery I got pregnant quickly.

My recovery after each birth was so fast that my husband would often have to remind me that I had just had a C-section and I probably shouldn't run down the stairs in such a hurry.

Bella is now five years old and Jacob is 18 months. They have not been immunized, but they have been having chiropractic adjustments since birth. Jacob has never been sick, and Bella has only been mildly sick once. I'm thankful I get to be a part of helping others have happy stories like mine at Erb Family Wellness. – Rebecca Gugeler

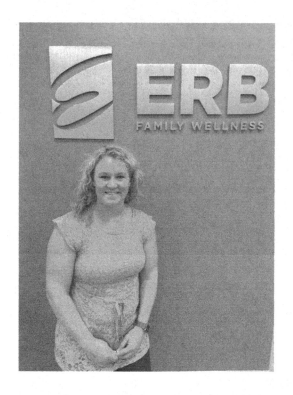

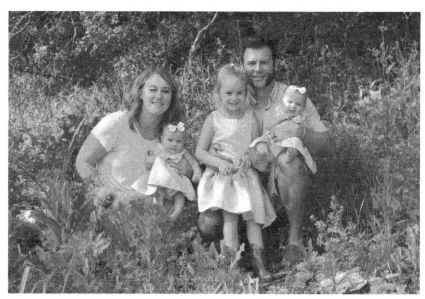

I had a friend who told me about Dr. Kimberly when she found out that we were trying to have a baby. I had already had four miscarriages by that time. My friend said the Erbs had a 100 percent success rate with their patients who were trying to get pregnant and carry to term.

We had already tried multiple avenues that ended in disappointment. We were doing IVF (in vitro fertilization) when we came to Erb Family Wellness. I was completely broken by that time. I had given up. I was on my knees. I thought that IVF would eliminate the problem that was thought to be my autoimmune disorder, but it didn't. Instead, we lost a baby the first time. The second time it didn't take, and I lost twins on the third try. That's when the doctor said, "We think, to give your babies the best chance at life you should get a surrogate."

Meanwhile, after the last try, Dr. Kimberly recommended metabolic testing. The test showed everything that I needed to do, every supplement I needed to take and exactly what I needed to eat. I followed the plan for 5 months. The first three were really intense, but after that I felt better. I was in the best shape of my life. I felt great. I looked great. I got up and I wasn't aching or hurting anymore.

The day after my birthday we transferred one of our embryos into the surrogate we chose. We prayed it would work. Then we went on vacation to get our minds off it all. I was a couple days late. So to be safe before enjoying a drink and scuba diving, I took a pregnancy test. I came out of a bathroom in Belize and announced to my husband that I was pregnant.

Our prayers before we left for vacation were also answered and our surrogate baby was born twelve days after I delivered. We got our twin babies after all!

I have no doubt that going to the Erbs helped me to get pregnant and to carry the baby. – Shandelyn Speake

# CHAPTER 9
# THE LITTLE ONES
# SUFFERING AT
# THE MERCY OF
# OUR INDOCTRINATION

"Start children off on the way they should go, and even
when they are old, they will not turn from it." Proverbs 22:6 NIV

The womb should be the safest place in the world for a little human. Sadly, in 2020 there have already been over 40,078,000 babies aborted and that number grows each second. But even for moms who are doing their best to protect and nourish their developing offspring the womb can still be a battleground. Babies are at the mercy of our choices, whether we're well informed or going with the flow of the Chemical Religion.

The unborn don't have a say. Who but us will protect them when the skin industry relies on dead babies' parts? The Bible calls us to stand up for the defenseless. "Speak up for people who cannot speak for themselves. Protect the rights of all who are helpless" (Proverbs 31:8 Good News Translation).

In this chapter, we're about to tell you all that *What to Expect When You're Expecting* didn't prepare you for so you can protect your developing baby.

## Surviving the Womb

When a woman discovers she's pregnant, she's filled with joy and anticipation. All she can think about is seeing her baby and the ultrasounds that have made it possible for her to catch glimpses before the ordained time.

"For you created my inmost being;
you knit me together in my mother's womb.
Your eyes saw my unformed body;
all the days ordained for me were written in your book
before one of them came to be."
Psalm 139:13,16 NIV

The womb is a secret place, and as much as we'd love to sneak a peek inside, it should remain hidden and protected. There's long been concerns for the safety of ultrasounds but without human testing the FDA has strongly discouraged (but not prohibited) the use of fetal ultrasound imaging use for creating keepsakes while also limiting the frequency levels. Shahram Vaezy, Ph.D., an FDA biomedical engineer warns, "Ultrasound can heat tissues slightly, and in some cases, it can also produce very small bubbles (cavitation) in some tissues."

Ultrasound administration is up 92% since 2004, according to new data reported by *The Wall Street Journal*. The American College of Obstetricians and Gynecologists only recommends getting one to two scans per low-risk pregnancy. Approximately 75% of pregnancies are considered low risk, yet most babies these days are currently being exposed to ultrasounds five or more times before they're delivered.

Ultrasounds have been known to cause cellular damage to developing babies and infertility in developing males. Prenatal exposure to low-frequency electromagnetic fields such as ultrasound, has been of particular concern. Some evidence shows an association with childhood leukemia, although studies have not consistently found a causal link between prenatal exposure to electromagnetic fields and birth defects, miscarriage or childhood leukemia until recently.

Research in the U.S. has been limited for ethical reasons of protecting human life. However, China's laws, which until recently enforced no more than one child to be born per family, allows them the opportunity to perform human studies. Their research proves "irrefutable evidence that human babies are always harmed in some, possibly subtle way, at minimum a trauma, from prenatal scans," stated the Healthy Home Economist. China conducted 50 studies including more than 2,700 pregnant women volunteering for the study to be performed on their soon-to-be-aborted babies. The fetuses were exposed to controlled diagnostic ultrasound and later analyzed by over 100 scientists.

Jim West is a medical critic and researcher who's made the Chinese causation studies available to us in the Western world through his book, *Diagnostic Ultrasound: A New Bibliography, Human Studies Conducted in Modern China*. The study indicates that, even at frequencies considered low by Western standards, prenatal ultrasound is a damaging form of medical radiation. The evidence strongly implies that prenatal ultrasound is responsible for the causation or initiation of the following conditions and disorders:

- Autism Spectrum Disorder
- ADHD
- Genetic damage, inheritable by future generations.
- Jaundice

- Childhood cancers, e.g., leukemia, lymphoma, brain, etc.
- Chorioamnionitis (inflammation of the maternal-fetal junction)
- Personality anomalies
- Ophthalmological diseases and various malformations
- Skin diseases such as eczema
- Allergies

West warns that ultrasound exposure "creates weaknesses in the unborn baby disabling its ability to overcome future stressors such as pharmaceuticals." It's similar to the perfect storm we talked about in Chapter Seven. A weakness is created in the womb, and when the newborn is injected with vaccines, some babies aren't able to recover and resist disease.

To ultrasound or not to ultrasound isn't the only question moms-to-be face. From the moment one discovers she's pregnant, discussions of natural birth verses induction, epidural (derived from cocaine) or cesarean are debated. Will she have a home birth or go to a birthing center?

She might choose to deliver in what has strangely come to be known as the "traditional" fashion, a hospital. Not that long ago all babies were born at home, but that began to change in the 1900's when the Chemical Religion initiated the medicalization of childbirth.

In a hospital, if a mom wants to have her baby naturally, she'll have to have a birth plan that's been discussed and agreed upon in advance with her doctor or she'll likely be subjected to epidural and abnormally intense birthing contractions from Pitocin. Inducing drugs have caused trauma to babies *and* moms, especially when the birth canal is being forced by a drug to push a baby out before it's been given time to expand and prepare through its natural process. The drug may also cause serious or life-threatening side effects in the newborn baby, including:

- Slow heartbeats or other abnormal heart rate

- Jaundice (which often requires baby to remain in the hospital after mom is released)

- Seizure

- Eye problems

- Breathing problems, muscle tone

Epidurals are another common practice that, without a birth plan, will likely be encouraged. They go hand in hand with Pitocin. If you have an epidural that numbs you in the part of your body necessary to the birthing process, your doctor will likely want you to be induced since you may be too numb to work with your natural contractions during delivery. This combination may put you and your baby at risk for forceps, vacuum, or C-section as the drugs can cause fetal heart rate changes indicating fetal distress.

Many families (like ours) had epidurals with their births. My wife had to have one with each of our children's deliveries because of an issue she had from an injury. Sometimes it's necessary, and we aren't here to judge anyone who has had one or who chooses to have one. We're here to inform you.

Waiting until you're in the vulnerable position of labor and delivery isn't the time to become informed and decide what kind of delivery experience you want. Learning the pros and cons of all your options empowers you to create a birth plan that protects your special birthing experience.

It's true that most women who've had an epidural praise the injection for its effectiveness in removing the pains of labor, but is pain relief the overall goal? Besides the women who suffer back pain every day since having had an epidural, many others complain about post-delivery experiences that they may not realize were a consequence of the drug. Epidurals also obstruct the hormones that aid in the experience such as oxytocin, known as the *love hormone*. Unmedicated mothers will experience the peak of their lifetime of the feel-good hormone at birth, but animal studies have shown difficulty bonding for epidural deliveries.

No one enjoys pain, but many mothers have experienced exhaustion from fussy, colicky babies. They've experienced lethargic babies who won't latch on to nurse. Hungry babies are fussy babies and fussy babies are very difficult to enjoy. The stories we hear from moms with epidural often sound like this, "I loved my epidural. I didn't feel anything. The room was serene." Then they transition to the first weeks with their baby and their tone changes. "I didn't get any sleep. No one wanted to hold my baby because he cried all the time." Or they shared stories of the first weeks waking their sleepy baby with cold, wet cloths just so they could get their tiny ones to take a few sips.

There are studies that validate and explain the experiences women have with their newborns:

- At one-month, epidural mothers described their babies as, "Less adaptable, more intense and more bothersome."

- 20 epidural babies compared with 20 unmedicated babies were found to be less alert and with less ability to orient for the first month of life.

- A large-population survey from Sweden found that use of an epidural was significantly associated with a low Apgar score at birth (the condition of the newborn at birth).

It's very likely these moms exchanged physical pain for emotional pain, while also putting themselves at risk for these issues:

- Cardiac arrest
- Maternal fever putting baby at risk for brain damage

- Respiratory depression
- Drop in blood pressure for up to half of all women with epidural
- Toxic reactions leading to paraplegia
- Inability to pass urine
- Shivering
- Sedation

- Postpartum hemorrhage
- Death 1 in 4,000 women (which is more than COVID, by the way)
- Blood clot (compressing spinal cord)
- Pruritus (itching)
- Nerve damage
- Nausea and vomiting

Our children are at the mercy of our choices. Every mother feels the weight of that burden, having to make tough decisions that affect them both. Here are some potential risks to babies that should be considered when deciding if an epidural is right for you:

- Higher rates of jaundice for epidural-exposed babies

- Fetal heartrate changes indicating lack of blood or oxygen

- Decrease in the oxygen supply to the baby's brain while also laying face up

- Poor tone

- Require resuscitation

- Seizures

- Loss of birth weight

- Four times more likely to be face up in final stages of labor

- Delay in Neurologic and Adaptive Capacity Score (NACS) from the drugs effect on newborns' neurobehavior

According to a Finnish survey, 67% of women injected with an epidural began supplementing or full formula-feeding within the first 12 weeks compared to 29% of nonepidural mothers. Low milk supply was also more often a complaint. The drugs stay in a newborn's system much longer and may be stored in tissues such as their liver and brain to be excreted more slowly. The emotional suffering that come from the drug's effects on babies may last for weeks forcing frustrated moms to give up on breastfeeding at their doctor's advice.

Moms receiving an epidural can have a pain-free birth but might not realize the satisfaction they're missing out on. The satisfaction of experiencing their body's strength. The pleasure of being fully connected to the power and intuition of their body uninhibited by drugs. The confidence of giving their newborn the best chance to thrive. If you're hoping to breastfeed, you can increase your chances for success and for a positive experience by having a drug-free labor and delivery.

As the World Health Organization comments, "epidural analgesia is one of the most striking examples of the *medicalization of normal birth*, transforming a physiological event into a medical procedure." Delivery is as natural and automatic to a woman's body as is breathing. You don't have to buy into the fear manufactured by the Chemical Religion.

## Cesarean Births

Speaking of medicalizing the birthing experience, cesarean births have nearly doubled worldwide since 2000. In that year there were 16 million caesarean births (or about 12% of all births). Childbirth experts say C-sections would account for about 10 to 15% of the babies delivered if they existed *only* for complications. The CDC and Prevention provisional data from 2019 show that the U.S. is still high with 31.7% of low-risk, first-time mothers having cesarean births.

As we've learned above, often times the epidural-Pitocin combo force complications, making it possible to further reduce that percentage. Why has the number skyrocketed? Besides increased drugs during labor and delivery, the natural process is being compromised for convenience.

C-sections are performed around doctors' schedules and are treated like a drive-thru—but without the fast-food rates. A C-section costs about 50% more than a typical vaginal delivery, making them a bit more tempting with respect to the bottom line. A woman's body is designed to know how and when to deliver a baby, but some women aren't getting the birth experience they hoped for because they're being encouraged to schedule a C-section around their doctor's vacation.

If you feel like you're being pressured into making choices for your delivery you're not comfortable with, it's okay to seek another opinion. Not all doctors practice with selfish motives. Or consider a midwife. Whatever you decide, remember it's you and your baby who will ultimately live with your choices.

Our goal isn't to tell you what to put on your birth plan. Every woman deserves to have the experience she desires when meeting her baby for the first time. No woman should judge another for her choices in the delivery room. And no woman should carry regrets. Like every other parent we are trying to do the best we can. We just want to share what we know so you can be informed before you go into labor.

## Is Breastfeeding Worth It?

The Chemical Religion has been downplaying the value of breastfeeding and causing confusion for many mothers. Some doctors tell moms not to bother, insisting there's a manmade alternative comparable to God's design.

Breastmilk is always changing to provide the nursing baby with what it needs to fight off sickness, sleep better, and to fill up growing babies' bellies.

A study on breastmilk took babies' blood, tested a little of mom's breast milk daily and found that it was different per child, per baby's needs and became more immune supportive daily for the needs of each infant. Mothers' milk changes to provide immune boosting for babies fighting sickness. When she's exposed to a virus Mom produces antibodies, which she passes to her infant through her milk. Formula cannot provide this benefit.

Human breastmilk has been shown to have a higher baseline level of immune cells when infants are exclusively breastfed. This may be why there was lower incidence of infections observed in the *breastfed only* group in a recent study. Immune cells in breast milk rapidly respond to either maternal or infant infection, suggesting a role in the protection of the mother as well as the infant. Believe me when I say you do not want to get sick when you have an infant! Trying to rest and recover with little ones who rely on you for their every need is difficult. Even worse is when mom and baby are both sick. Having a built-in immune response to protect both is a huge incentive for breastfeeding. It is yet another benefit that packaged milk cannot provide.

Mother's milk also changes from day to night. Evening milk contains more serotonin and other elements to help babies sleep. It changes *during* each feeding. The milk gets more filling towards the end. When nursing, feed your baby beyond your milks first course "appetizer," and give baby time to get to the "meatier" part of your milk.

Let us assure you that your breastmilk is *liquid gold*! It's worth the effort. We've talked about the complications that can occur for moms desiring to breastfeed their babies. We know it can be hard for some initially, so here's an encouraging list of benefits to help you stay motivated on hard days. Do the best you can and stick with it. Focus on the intimate time it gives you to share with your baby, and remember this:

## The Benefits of Giving Liquid Gold to Babies

- Stronger immune systems
- Less gastro issues
- Fewer colds and respiratory
- Fewer ear infections
- Fewer case of bacterial meningitis
- Lower rates of respiratory illness
- Lower rates of infant mortality
- Less likelihood of becoming obese later in childhood
- Fewer instances of allergies, eczema, and asthma
- Less illness overall and less hospitalization
- Fewer childhood cancers, including leukemia and lymphomas
- Lower rates of SIDS
- Fewer instances of Crohn's disease
- Better vision
- Fewer speech and orthodontic problems
- Fewer cavities
- Lower risk of type I and II diabetes
- Improved brain maturation
- Greater immunity to infection
- Less likely to develop rheumatoid arthritis and lupus
- Less likely to develop heart disease in adulthood
- Lower risk of multiple sclerosis
- Lower rates of pre-and postmenopausal breast cancers

## The Benefits of Breastfeeding for Moms:

- Lower risk of breast cancer
- Lower risk of ovarian cancer
- Lower risk of rheumatoid arthritis and lupus
- Lower chance of diabetes
- Less osteoporosis with age
- Less cardiovascular disease

- **Parents have up to six times less absenteeism from work since their babies aren't sick as often**
- Less endometriosis

- Less hypertension: it decreases blood pressure

Breastfeeding is convenient for travel, way less expensive than the man-made alternative and a lot healthier for baby. One popular baby formula brand lists corn syrup and sugar as the first and second ingredients. These products are dangerously genetically modified, meaning that infants are ingesting pesticides and GMOs from their formula. The third ingredient in this particular product is milk protein isolate, which is milk. Nonorganic milk also contains high levels of GMOs and pesticides as do all soy-based products in case you're considering a vegetarian option. It's unfathomable that such harmful ingredients can be found in food for our tiniest and most helpless humans.

Reading the loud marketing on the front of packaging rather than the small print on the back label is deceptive. Companies can get away with telling you what you want to hear on the front, but the ingredients will tell a more truthful story if you know what to look for. Better yet, breastmilk doesn't come with labels and marketing. Mom is in control of what she eats, thus what she feeds her baby.

In Chapter Three we talked more about the dangers of glyphosate, but our little ones' livers are less developed and incapable of detoxing the way an adult liver can. Their bodies are much more sensitive to the long-term effects and yet foods designed for them contain some of the highest levels of this poison.

"There is no acceptable number of herbicides or GMOs that should be in a baby's diet," warned Dr. Michelle Perro, board-certified in Pediatrics with more than 30 years of experience. If formula becomes necessary, she implores her patients to use an organic source.

Baby foods containing grains such as rice, wheat or oats tested positive for residues of glyphosate. The levels found in well-known baby foods that include grains in the ingredients averaged 14.3 parts per billion, which is 143 times higher than the amount allowed in European drinking water.

The marketing is everywhere. The indoctrination is deeply ingrained into our society targeting our kids at the earliest of ages. (Why put sugar in baby formula?) Get them addicted to the cancer-fostering-substance, sugar in their cereals which are also full of glyphosate and they've got them. The addicted throw fits when they don't get what they want even if what they want is deadly. We have to stay informed so that we aren't unintentionally spoon-feeding sickness to our young ones.

The food industry's propaganda enforced by the FDA's food pyramid nonsense made for acceptable practices such as preschools and church nurseries handing out high GMO fishy crackers served with bleached white milk to our kids. They do this without thinking it is necessary to get our permission. A taste for the toxic products is introduced to our kids and soon those snacks will be expected to make their way into our grocery carts!

Whether it's infant formula (the only meals babies consume all day) or in baby and toddler foods, or in those horrendous school lunches that should be ashamed for claiming to be healthy; exchanging just one GMO meal a day for a healthy organic meal could prevent or reverse health issues such as we discussed in Chapter Eight for infertility. Imagine how changing your little ones' diet can impact their health and give them a healthier start in life!

### How Well-Baby Checkups Make for Sick Babies

In Chapter One we provided a lot of facts discrediting the vaccine myth. In this chapter we'll just add a few refreshers as it pertains to what has become common concerns in this age for our little ones. SIDS, asthma and allergies, ear infections, and learning disabilities (such as autism) come to mind. These can all be linked to those well-baby checkups where you'll be expected to subject your infants and toddlers to vaccinations. You'll be assured they're safe but if you resist, your pediatrician will manipulate you with fear to comply. In most cases they are only regurgitating what they've been taught by information provided them by pharmaceutical companies. Remember Big Pharma's mantra? *"The benefits outweigh the risk."* There's plenty of evidence discrediting the benefits, but the superpowers have all the money they need to keep it hidden. Try searching Google for "vaccine risks" and all that will surface are what pharmaceutical companies want you to know. They all say the same thing as if rehearsed. We've dug deeper to bring you the truth.

In 1975 Japan raised the minimum age of vaccination from two months to two years. Crib death, infantile seizures, meningitis, and other infectious diseases in infants virtually disappeared. Japan went from seventeenth in infant mortality to first place, acquiring the lowest incidence of infant mortality in the world! However, they had a new crop of neurologically damaged two-year-old's after vaccinations, providing further proof that the risks outweigh the benefits. In fact, it seems to indicate the *lack* of benefits.

In contrast, American babies receive their first shot at birth, and we have a distressingly high infant mortality rate! Nearly twenty countries are better than the U.S., yet we rave about our "excellent" healthcare.

Asthma is a terrifying affliction both for the child who can't breathe and for the parent who is trying to comfort their child. It's yet another disease that has been on the rise since the evolution of child vaccines. Could there be a correlation?

- A New Zealand study published in *Epidemiology* studied immunized children and those who were not. Of the immunized children, 23.1% had asthma and 30% had other allergic illnesses. **None (that's 0%) of the non-immunized children had asthma or other allergic illness.**

- In another study there was 1 case of asthma out of the 91 who had no vaccinations at all.

- Between 15 and 20% of American school children are considered learning disabled, with minimal brain dysfunction directly caused by vaccine damage. In fact, vaccination before one year of age was associated with increased odds of developmental delays, *asthma* and ear infections. The odds increased as more vaccines were received.

- Vaccinated children showed higher odds of being diagnosed with pneumonia, otitis media (middle ear inflammation), allergies, and neurodevelopmental disorders.

- Hurwitz and Morgenstern reported an association between diphtheria–tetanus–pertussis (DTP) and tetanus toxoid vaccination and allergy symptoms and could not rule out a relationship with asthma.

- 10.69% of children immunized (with pertussis) got asthma

- Children vaccinated with DPPT (or MMR) had **14 times more asthma** and **9.4 times more eczema** than non-vaccinated children

- "**80%** of the cases of measles are contracted **in vaccinated people**."

When our son Zac was three years old his peers got the MMR shot, which includes measles vaccine. Zac caught measles from his contact with them. He ran a 104.5-degree temperature for 12 hours then was covered in bumps. It's never easy seeing your children sick, but Zac was unlike his peers. He suffered through the measles naturally, which strengthened his immune system and in 24 hours the worst was over. He was fully recovered from the rash in just ten days. Many of his peers were vaccinated against measles and have suffered allergies ever since.

Harris Coulter, Ph.D., encourages that, "Contracting and overcoming childhood diseases are part of a developmental process that actually helps develop a healthy, robust, adult immune system able to meet the challenges that inevitable encounters with virus and bacteria will present later on."

The risk of a serious vaccine reaction may be 100 times greater than the risk of hepatitis B. Asthma, diabetes, autism and attention deficit/hyperactivity disorder have increased greatly since the introduction of many new vaccines according to Jane Orient, M.D., Executive Director Association of American Association of Physicians and Surgeons. Keeping in mind how few vaccine injuries are reported, the following are the number of reports to VAERS of some conditions and symptoms occurring shortly after Hepatitis B vaccination:

- Multiple Sclerosis 50

- Guillain Barre' Syndrome 113

- Myelitis/Encephalomyelitis 108

- Optic Neuritis 67

- Paralysis 342

- Ataxia 129

- Confusion 51

- Hearing loss 32

- Autism 121

We know we have listed a lot of facts and studies here, but there are so many more. It's important that we present evidence to back up the truth we are telling. Vaccinations are not the cure.

- The number of injuries and deaths from the Hepatitis B vaccine are **20 times greater** than that from the disease

- Hepatitis B vaccine is linked to lupus and multiple sclerosis (MS).

- In a study involving Korean children who were all vaccinated against hepatitis B, a significantly higher asthma incidence was seen among children.

- **Nearly 90% of the total decline in mortality** (scarlet fever, diphtheria, whooping cough, and measles) between 1860 and 1965 **occurred before the introduction of antibiotics and widespread immunization."**

Do the benefits really outweigh the risks? Besides all the evidence stacked against vaccinations, experts encourage us that contracting and overcoming childhood diseases build a healthy, robust, adult immune system that can overcome future viruses and bacteria.

When we were kids our moms would take us for play dates with friends who had chicken pox so we could build up an immunity to it. It's unbelievable to us that now there's a shot for that, too! Our natural immune system is more powerful when it's exposed and given the opportunity to strengthen itself. Mom was smart to give our bodies an opportunity to grow stronger with exposure versus "protecting" us from viruses and inadvertently weakening our immunity.

**Chiropractic is the Redemption of Healthcare**

Not all ear infections, allergies, and asthma come from shots. Along with colic, gas, reflux, and bed wetting they can be corrected with diet and spinal adjustments. Birth subluxation is a common factor in fussy babies. This freaks a lot of moms out, but babies need spinal adjustments too. Yes, even newborns! Think about what those little guys go through; forced down a tiny tunnel, then coming out headfirst without neck muscles to support their bobble! Although God's design for birth is perfect (with 80% of babies born without spinal issues) early chiropractic care can catch any subluxation before it becomes a problem. Even babies born with the most perfectly curved spine will benefit from the immune boost a spinal adjustment gives.

We adjust babies all the time in our office and the only effects are happier babies with healthier immune systems.

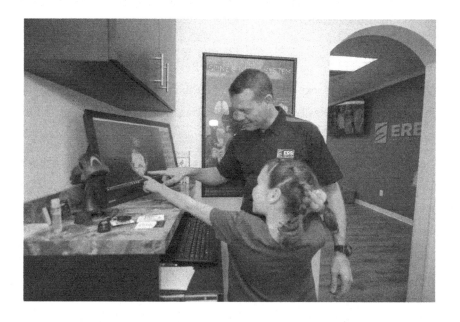

Pediatricians can offer surgery and an array of meds that may mask the symptoms of reflux, gas, allergies and asthma but all drugs force the body into compliance as though it were taking it hostage. Working with your child's natural immune system only has positive results. We can help you find the kind of doctors who know how to help you and your growing family thrive. Chiropractors are the reemerging heroes in these dark days of Big Pharma and a corrupt food industry bloating our government with their underhanded methods. Chiropractic is the redemption of healthcare!

## Has the School System Been Indoctrinated to Indoctrinate?

Besides the "well-baby" checkups, the pressure to conform hits hardest when enrolling your children in school. The school nurse looks at you sideways when you explain that you won't be updating your student's shot records. They threaten that your kids won't be allowed to start school. Then they look down on you when you give them the government affidavit that permits admittance. Some parents fear the system more than the vaccines potential side effects and decide to take their chances.

Many teachers pressure parents to put active students, especially boys, on ADHD meds. Without the facts, some parents appease the lazy teaching method. Zombie-like students sitting quietly in their seats, void of personality make for a quiet day in the classroom. Drug induced compliance seems more like a psych ward than a healthy learning environment. Teaching methods that allow for movement, exploration, and creative expression can be challenging, but they make the classroom feel like a safe place for individuality and learning. One pill leads to another, and if ADHD meds are prescribed, drugged kids have entered the Chemical Religion system. We must stand against the propaganda, against the pressure and remove our kids from the cycle of sugar addiction, medication and sickness.

We've experienced teachers who take liberties in the classroom, contributing to the indoctrination of our youth. When Zac was in first grade, I began getting reports every day of his bad behavior in class. This went on for five or six weeks! I was getting on to my son whose apparent behavior was embarrassing me.

The teacher called me one day and described Zac as "a continual disruption in class and disrespectful." She said he was out of control. When I probed a little more into what was going on, I discovered they were doing a cancer research project in class. The teacher was showing six-year-old children's videos of bald kids on chemotherapy. The students were supposed to write letters and draw pictures to be given to the kids with cancer. I'm sure it must've been scary for some in the classroom to see kids their own age fighting for their lives. They were suddenly faced with a question interrupting their innocence, "Can this happen to me?"

I was angry that I had not been notified for my consent, but I decided to give my son the opportunity to use his voice instead of giving her a piece of my mind. I asked his teacher, "Have you ever asked Zac what he thinks of the project?" We had taught our children the principles of health and healing that we're giving you in this book. He had seen sick people made well in our office before he could even talk. So, when his teacher asked him his opinion he responded, "I just think all these kids should learn about chiropractic and nutrition."

Zac did his first doctors report at six years old in front of his peers. He presented facts about how to find true health through chiropractic and proper nutrition. By the end of the class every student wanted to be a chiropractor. The teacher was livid because that's what sometimes happens when ingrained beliefs are challenged. Sometimes truth embarrasses us. It disrupts us. The truth can be an offense, but there's wisdom in humility. Admitting to ourselves that we were wrong allows us to grow and be better. We're responsible for what we know.

**"Speak for those who cannot speak; seek justice for all those on the verge of destruction." Proverbs 31:8 ISV**

Another tragic example of children without a voice and no one to speak up for them is in the foster care system. These kids immediately become a part of the Chemical Religion's system, where not even an M.D. can rescue them. We've known kids who became violent after being prescribed mind-altering drugs. Even with a medical doctor's recommendation the kids had no choice but to stay on the meds that further endangered those caring for them and endangered themselves. Anti-depressants are given to 95% of kids in the foster care program. In Chapter Seven we showed you the dangers and the risks associated with mental illness meds and debunked the "chemical imbalance" theory pushed by the Chemical Religion. These children and our children need someone to speak up for them.

The attack on the vulnerable begins in the womb and continues through every stage of our children's lives. We can protect them by learning the truth and teaching our children to avoid the flow of chemicals and toxins that most are caught up in. We use our voice until they are old enough to use theirs to stand up for themselves.

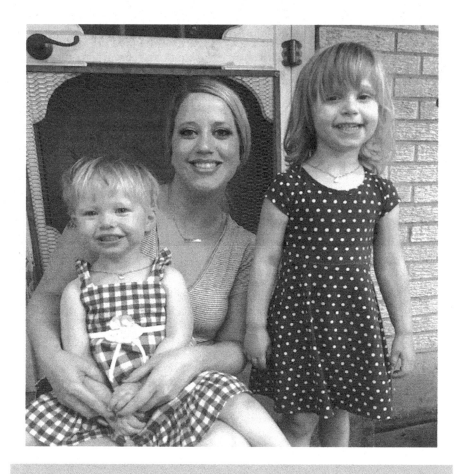

Thank you, Dr. David, for caring for my little one!!!

For any pregnant mama's out there or existing parents with kids that have never heard about the benefits of having your children adjusted by a doctor who corrects subluxation, come to the Erbs to see just how simple, quick and painless an adjustment is, even on an infant. My daughter was only 4 days old!

Many parents don't understand that pediatricians don't have the expertise to determine if your child has any subluxations in the neck or spine. Most infants have some type of subluxation due to being in the womb and/or from childbirth. These small subluxations gone untreated can lead to sickness and health issues.

I posted a testimony last year about my other daughter Arya's clogged tear duct, that never cleared up on its own. I had NOT had her examined after birth by Dr. David. When my normal pediatrician recommended we put tubes in her eye at 8 months, I knew there had to be a more reasonable and simple solution. After 2-3 adjustments with Dr. David, her tear duct completely cleared, and we have been getting her adjusted about every 2-3 weeks since. She's never had ear infections, or any major sickness. Anytime she's had a fever we just get her adjusted more often and do not use any fever medicine. I think she's had a fever twice the past 19 months. She has been one healthy kid overall.

If you are the type of parent that is looking for alternative care, are tired of taking your kids to urgent care and pumping them with antibiotics or over the counter meds, then reach out to these doctors!

Lastly, I was adjusted my entire pregnancy and can say I had a very healthy pregnancy. My contractions started at 4:30 pm on Monday afternoon, we arrived at the hospital at 1:30 am with strong contractions and at 4:13 am I had baby Thea. When I arrived at the hospital, I was only dilated to a 4.5 but in an hour and a half, I progressed to a 9 and was ready to push. Thanks to the good Lord I was able to have Thea naturally, with no epidural and had a water birth. This is quite the opposite experience I had with my first pregnancy. I was two weeks past my due date and had to be induced. It took 36 hours before Arya arrived. I begged for an epidural close to the end because I was so exhausted from the unnatural contractions from the Pitocin I was given. Both births ended with a healthy baby. Praise God! I will confess that I 100% believe the outcome of my second birth is due to the positive effects of being adjusted during my pregnancy.

All women are different, and this post is not to shame anyone else's childbirth story if you had an outcome less favorable than mine. I just wanted to share my testimony so that if you ever wanted to consider alternative care outside your OBGYN, keep an open mind and heart on the topic of chiropractic care. Your mind will be blown at all the benefits you never considered were possible with chiropractic care. I hope someone can benefit from me sharing this! – Haven Savage

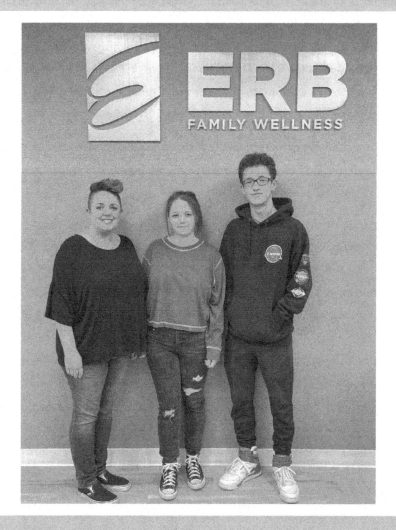

A friend referred me to Dr. David in 2008. I had suffered for about five years with neuropathy in my hands and feet. I needed help. The doctors

kept putting me on multiple meds that didn't work. Some of them even made me gain weight.

One of the first things Dr. David asked me was if I used Splenda. I told him I used it because I heard it was healthier than sugar. After just two adjustments and giving up Splenda, I was symptom free and off all meds.

My son was two years old when we started going to Erb Family Wellness. I believe he had been vaccine injured after a doctor gave him a flu shot at nine months old. That night he started turning blue. Since that time until we started going to the Erbs, he was in and out of hospitals for lung related issues. My son was diagnosed with asthma before he was even a year old. We spent weeks in multiple hospitals with him where he almost died a few times. I stopped getting my kids vaccinated after that.

Dr. David started adjusting my son and teaching me about fevers. He would say, "Fevers are a good thing." I was nervous when my son was running a fever. We took him to get adjusted and his fever was immediately gone within ten minutes after the adjustment. I was a believer!

My kids are 18- and 15-years-old now and they are very healthy. They never get sick, and my son no longer needs asthma medications. – Jennifer Arteaga

# CHAPTER 10
# FEARFULLY AND WONDERFULLY MADE: HAVE WE FORGOTTEN?

"You made all the delicate, inner parts of my body and knit me together in my mother's womb." Psalms 139: 14-16 NLT

We love our teenagers, bless their hearts, but raising teens in a culture that has been taught to self-diagnose and self-medicate through pharmaceuticals, vaping, and alcohol hasn't been easy. Even marijuana is becoming an acceptable method for coping with life's ups and downs. What ever happened to Nancy Reagans slogan, *"Just say 'no'"*? Unfortunately, a lot has changed since she simplified the choice to refuse drugs.

### What's Opened the Door to Teen Drug Use?

We were at a parent teacher orientation where all the parents were being asked to bring in a bag of candy. The teacher wanted to use it as bribes to get kids to answer questions and stay on task. That's how our son Zac got his first cavity! He was given suckers every day and would hold it in his mouth against his teeth. There's an even bigger problem than rotting teeth. Sugar is an addictive drug that gives an energy boost followed by a drop in blood sugar that causes sleepiness and lack of focus. We're teaching our kids that they need help getting their brains to work instead of teaching them discipline. We could be emphasizing nutrition and getting enough sleep so that they'll say "no" to sugar and say "no" to the other drugs they'll soon face to stay focused in class. (See Chapter Three for more on sugar.)

When we were growing up, we only had TV and radio to influence us, but today's youth are being fed what to believe on Snapchat, Tic Tok, Instagram, and memes. The manipulating images are all over what teens stare at most, their phones! Actors in adds with sad faces pop a pill and suddenly happy butterflies flying amidst the sun's rays brainwashing our kids into believing happiness must be prescribed.

Teens have been wired to believe we're broken requiring chemicals to survive. Forgetting that humans have been created in the image of God, some have even begun to worship the medications over the God who said we're fearfully and wonderfully made. They'd rather have a diagnosis from a doctor than seek out healing from the Creator.

Many young people think there are cures for the things that make us human, like our ability to experience life through our emotions. They look for ways to overcome our God-given need for rest. Big Pharma and the food industry offer them a chance to be superhuman, but it may cost them their health, their freedom and eventually their life.

Stimulants such as caffeine, nicotine in vaping and Adderall have become popular among the youth of today. You may not see an athlete on the sidelines sipping a cup of coffee, but energy drinks such as Monsters, Bangs, and Red Bulls are becoming an epidemic among aspiring stars.

The energy drink business is a $3 billion industry targeting teenagers and young adults. From 2004 to 2009, energy drink sales increased 240% while the emergency room visits for caffeine overdoses also increased. In 2009, 56% of the 13,114 overdose ER visits were kids between the ages of 12-19. By 2011, the energy drinks' marketing had become so successful in convincing consumers to "tear into" a can that the number grew to 20,783 visits!

One popular brand advertises, "Gives you wings whenever you need them," suggesting their product offers a second wind. Students and young athletes buy into the marketing as they chug the **whole** can. Many brands contain *two* servings of caffeine with other hidden caffeine forms and stimulants. Their combination of caffeine, guarana, and taurine can cause other more severe health risks such as:

- Increased risk of strokes
- Blood clots
- Heart attacks
- Cardiac arrhythmias
- Kidney failure
- Death

Some young consumers have not been given the second wind they were promised. Their final breaths came after drinking the dangerous beverage they were made to believe would give them wings.

Monster is linked to deaths and heart attacks in a growing number of people who believe the drink will make them better. The labels are misleading. Consumers aren't warned of how the product's other ingredients stimulate and stress the heart in combination with the caffeine listed or how caffeine increases urine production putting them at risk for dehydration. They aren't warned of the addictive nature of caffeine regarding tolerance which increases with regular consumption and the dependency that it creates causing withdrawals such as headaches, brain fog and depression.

Even if the labels made clear the dangers of energy drinks, we've seen from pharmaceuticals that people are more convinced by marketing than they are by warning labels, especially our impressionable youth. Young people often think they're invincible. Every parent of teens can attest to the fact that teenagers aren't exactly known for using good judgment all the time. So, when another cup of joe doesn't work to give teens an edge, they resort to adding another energy beverage. When that stops doing the trick because their body's grown use to the dosage, they start looking for what's next without considering the consequences. Whether through marketing or from peers willing to sell them a pill from their bottle, they may get turned on to the "smart pill."

### "Smart" Pills

The competition to get into college and to do well has our youth seeking out whatever they can find to make them stand out. They see the ads for miracle pills that'll keep them focused and awake with no need to waste time on silly human things like sleep and food.

Close to 50 million prescription stimulant drugs such as Adderall (amphetamine-dextroamphetamine) were dispensed in 2011 to treat symptoms of attention deficit hyperactivity disorder, or ADHD. These drugs may be more socially acceptable, but don't be fooled: they're in the same family as methamphetamine ("meth") and are as addictive. Sometimes my wife and I wonder where the lines are between drug dealer and pediatrician.

Adderall, known by kids as a "smart drug," is being passed out by some doctors like candy, making it easy for kids to pass pills out to their friends who don't have a prescription. Most parents would never serve up a line of meth and a snorting straw with their child's breakfast, but many give them a little pill with the same effects before sending them off to school. With good intentions, they're naively turning their children into addicts.

Even students are beginning to believe they can't even take a test without their pills! In fact, a study at the University of Kentucky found that 30% of its students had abused an ADHD stimulant drug like Adderall at some point as a possible "study enhancer." Kids are literally praising these pills and giving up their freedom in exchange for an addiction that they believe will give them a brighter future. They may actually be laying their lives down to a false god.

Adderall's side effects include:

- Lethargy
- Sleep disruption
- High blood pressure
- Stroke
- Depression
- Bipolar disorder
- Heart disease
- Sleep difficulties
- Inability to concentrate
- Lack of motivation
- Depression
- Irritability
- Physical damage to the brain and internal systems and organs
- Fatigue
- Aggression
- Thoughts of suicide
- Mood swings
- Paranoia
- Hallucinations
- Anxiety
- Panic attacks
- Aggressive or hostile behavior
- Weight loss
- Headaches
- Tremors
- Constipation

Other side effects of abusing Adderall long-term include:

- Dizziness
- Abdominal pain
- Weight loss
- Insomnia
- Dry mouth
- Heart palpitations
- Tremors
- Trouble breathing
- Hyperactivity
- Feeling jittery or "on edge"

Even more dangerous than taking this drug is combining it with alcohol. The deadly mixture of depressant with stimulant counter acts the effects of each causing over consumption. But alcohol isn't the only depressant teens are bowing to.

## Rx Euphoria

Pharma created the drug MDMA to treat anxiety and depression, but it was outlawed by the United States in 1985. Since then, it's gone underground, now referred to by teens as the popular club drug they call "Molly" or "Ecstasy." They use it for its euphoric and slightly hallucinogenlike experiences that numb them to their reality.

Xanax, another popular drug among the youth, is prescribed for anxiety, panic disorders, and anxiety associated with depression. The younger generation hasn't been taught how to effectively manage the day-to-day stresses in life through planning, communication, healthy meditation, diet and exercise. Instead, the natural fears that we all struggle to overcome are now considered disorders in need of a pill.

Xanax doesn't cure anything. It doesn't offer tools for how to overcome anxiety. It's in the class of psychoactive drugs next to Valium that offer a euphoric feeling. It's a highly addictive drug that alters the functions of the brain and the central nervous system that comes with a whole new set of side effects such as:

- Memory problems
- Dementia
- Alzheimer's
- Drowsiness
- Fatigue
- Dizziness
- Unusual risk-taking behavior
- Difficulty concentrating
- Sexual dysfunction
- Depression
- Slow or shallow breathing
- Respiratory arrest
- Addiction
- Suicidal thoughts
- Headaches
- Decreased inhibitions in dangerous situations
- Death
- Seizures

So, we give teens who are already known for not making good choices a pill that "decreases inhibitions in dangerous situations." Really?

Xanax is to blame for about 30% of overdose-related deaths each year. When a patient tries to get off the drug, the severe withdrawals have been known to cause deadly seizures. The Chemical Religion doesn't want us to get free. It wants to hook our youth and have customers for life. It's been exposed for making false statements with no apology for the deaths their products have caused. After the opioid crisis, I'm not quite sure how anyone can still put their trust in them.

### They Lied Before, What Makes You Think They Won't Lie Again?

The youth of our society have been brainwashed to believe pain, whether emotional or physical, is a sickness requiring medical advice. When a young woman has menstrual cramps, she's given birth control pills. If a teen is stressed about his grades, he's prescribed Xanax to calm his nerves. "Why would a patient swallow a poison because he is ill or take that which would make a well man sick?" asked L.F. Kebler, M.D. When did pain become a disease?

In the mid-1990s the American Pain Society along with other groups began to push doctors to include pain in their vital sign checks along with temperature, breathing rate, blood pressure, and pulse rate. Until then, wanting to protect their patients from possible addiction, M.D.s were reluctant to prescribe opioids. But with dollar signs in their eyes, pharmaceutical companies began to successfully market their products to doctors as having a low risk for addiction. What business wouldn't want their customers to become addicted to their products! That's more customers for life since the addicted are willing to do anything, even harm themselves to get another fix. And Big Pharma is willing to do anything for another dollar.

Worldwide, about 350,000 people die every year from opioid use. One survey showed that one of every eight high school seniors said they'd used prescription opioids for nonmedical reasons.

The U.S. Senate Finance Committee began an investigation in search of documentation of financial and other inappropriate links between the makers of the top-prescribed narcotic painkillers and pain organizations such as Purdue Pharma, Endo Pharmaceuticals and Johnson & Johnson, as well as the American Pain Foundation, American Academy of Pain Medicine, American Pain Society, Wisconsin Pain & Policy Studies Group and the Center for Practical Bioethics.

As concerns grew over the abuse of opioids, it became clear there was an unholy union between Big Pharma and the so called "not-for-profit" group. Pushing the Chemical Religion's greedy plan, the American Pain Foundation received 90% of its $5 million funding from the drug and medical-device industry in 2010. Further deception came through the patient guides and other publications that exaggerated the painkillers' benefits while making light of their risks.

"When it comes to these highly addictive painkillers, improper relationships between pharmaceutical companies and the organizations that promote their drugs can put lives at risk," Senator Max Baucus of Montana said in a prepared statement.

Dr. Andrew Kolodny, chairman of psychiatry at Maimonides Medical Center in Brooklyn, N.Y., and president of Physicians for Responsible Opioid Prescribing warned, "These groups, these pain organizations ... helped usher in an epidemic that's killed 100,000 people by promoting aggressive use of opioids. What makes this especially disturbing is that despite overwhelming evidence that their effort created a public health crisis, they're continuing to minimize the risk of addiction."

Opioids shouldn't be taken lightly. They come with big risks:

- Addiction

- A 40% to 60% higher risk of suicidal ideation

- Habitual users are twice as likely to attempt suicide

But for many leaders in the Chemical Religion, opioids come with much to gain. Corrupt doctors and drug stores worked together to fill prescriptions. Lawsuits are holding drug distributors and well-known pharmacies accountable though the profits they made will likely outweigh the compensation they will owe.

In just five years, top pharmaceutical companies spent **$13,048,700,000** in settlements for fraudulent marketing practices and the promotion of medicines for uses that were not approved by the FDA. That doesn't include the **$110,000,000** Bayer paid to Yaz pill patients we talked about in Chapter Eight. Even after these enormous settlements some companies have already been caught committing the crime again and have had to pay more millions.

Chemical Religion evangelists lie. Purdue Pharma pled guilty to federal criminal charges that it misled regulators, physicians and consumers about Oxycontin's risk of addiction. The evidence of this industry's greed at the expense of trusting patients is undeniable.

In 2017 Health and Human Services declared a nationwide public health emergency for the epidemic and invested almost $900 million to combat the damage done by the deceptions of the medical industry. America paid for the greed of the corrupt industry in lives and in tax dollars, while Big Pharma doesn't seem to be afraid of paying out millions or billions in settlements. They're making so much money, it's a drop in the bucket. Besides, settling outside of court ensures they won't be fully exposed thus maintaining the trust of M.D.s and consumers.

### How Do They Get Away with It?

Do you ever wonder how they get away with such atrocities in our first world country with a government that was established *for* the people?

The New York Times reported that about a quarter of every dollar spent in the United States goes to the FDA whose purpose as defined by their website is: "The Food and Drug Administration is responsible for protecting the public health by ensuring the safety, efficacy, and security of human and veterinary drugs, biological products, and medical devices; and by ensuring the safety of our nation's food supply, cosmetics, and products that emit radiation." But is that what they're doing?

Since the mid-1990s, studies have exposed that around 85 to 90% of new drugs don't offer any clinical advantages for users although, there's definitely been monetary advantages for the medical industry from them. Regardless of the lack of innovative meds coming out, in 2014, the FDA expedited approval for 46% of fresh on the market pharmaceuticals making them the fastest regulatory agency in the world for new drugs and approving 96% of all never-before-marketed pharmaceuticals.

In 2016 the House passed the 21st Century Cures Act, backed by Big Pharma, by a 344-77 vote that unleashed drug companies to push their drugs to patients faster with less true testing.

Harvard professor Daniel Carpenter described the legislation as "'The 19th Century Frauds Act', it enables device companies to use anecdotes as valid, sufficient scientific evidence that a medical device works; drug companies to submit animal studies in lieu of clinical — human — trials to prove antibiotics' efficacy and safety; and doctors to be paid by pharmaceutical companies for certain incentives without disclosing them."

So much for the FDA upholding "safety and efficacy." How can they have the people's best interests when they're pushing Big Pharma's agenda along with the House of Representatives? If the government won't protect us, we have to start protecting ourselves.

If a convicted murderer said he had a pill that would save your child's life, would you entrust your child to his care? Pharmaceutical companies have confessed to intentionally lying about their products to increase sells. They confessed to releasing products that had not yet been approved nor had they been thoroughly tested. They've been convicted of pushing pills for diseases that the pills were not formulated to treat. People have died from their products! Why are we still subjecting ourselves to their practices? Are we laying ourselves on their alters to be sacrificed to their god?

**More Lies. More Loss.**

The Chemical Religion tells us to get our kids the HPV vaccine. They tell us it will protect our teens from contracting the sexually transmitted disease that causes cancer and can hinder fertility. They'll never admit guilt when our daughters become infertile or develop cancer from the injection. They offer expensive pills and treatments instead—as long as we keep trusting them.

We had a young lady come to our office for thermography. She was in her early 20's and her PAP revealed she had the HPV virus. The sweet girl had been vaccinated (though she wasn't sexually active) and yet she now had the virus. She got it from the vaccine! We have to stop believing the lies. (For more about the HPV vaccine see Chapter Eight.)

**Beautiful, But Suicidal**

My wife and I have had to overcome things just like everyone else. We've gone through health scares that made us search for answers for ourselves before bringing the healing to others.

I had a happy childhood with a great family. My mom showed her love every morning with fresh cinnamon rolls for breakfast before school and pie for dinner after football. It was literally a sweet life, until I got hit hard with cystic acne all over my body. I wanted to hide, but when you're a football star you have to take showers, exposing yourself to your entire team. I felt ugly and embarrassed.

My parents and I sought help from our local doctor when the cysts would get so bad my eyes were swollen shut. I spent a lot of time on antibiotics to control infection from the open wounds. But my life changed when he prescribed Accutane and almost suddenly my skin was clear.

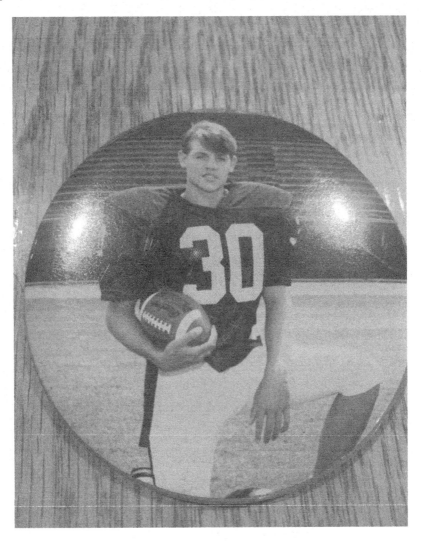

It seemed that all my problems were solved. I was voted best looking my senior year, but I started having dark thoughts about killing myself. I had to figure out another solution.

I realized that my diet needed to change (sorry Mom) and that my gut flora was destroyed from all the antibiotics. I got off Accutane after meeting my wife and, with her help and encouragement, I began to heal my body so that I could be acne free. It wasn't easy and it wasn't fast, but it may have saved my life.

Accutane was marketed by Hoffmann-La Roche until 2009. Roche removed it from the U.S. market after juries awarded millions of dollars to its consumers who suffered inflammatory bowel disease side-effect. It then became generic and is now marketed under many brand names worldwide.

The list of common to rare side effects is too long to add them all here:

- 10% or more had increased red blood cell sedimentation rate (up to 40%).

- 1% to 10% had a low number of neutrophils in blood (a type of white blood cell made in the bone marrow that help your body fight infection and bacteria anemia).

- 10% or more had increased blood triglycerides/hypertriglyceri-demia (up to 30%).

- 1% to 10% increased blood cholesterol/hyperlipidemia a high level of lipids/ fats in blood which include cholesterol or tri-glycerides which increase risk for heart disease, heart attack and stroke.

- Increased blood glucose/alterations in blood sugar levels, decreased high density lipoprotein.

- 1% to 10% Arthralgia/severe arthralgia, back pain/severe back pain, myalgia/severe myalgia with or without elevated creatine phosphokinase (CPK) levels.

- Rhabdomyolysis the breakdown of muscle tissue that leads to the release of muscle fiber contents into the blood. These substances are harmful to the kidney and often cause kidney damage, sometimes leading to hospitalization. Death has sometimes occurred, especially in patients undertaking vigorous physical activity.

Lab tests on 13,772 Kaiser Permanente patients taking isotretinoin in the brand Accutane or in three generic versions were studied. The patients being treated from March 1995 to September 2002 were between 13 to 50 years old. The findings were published in the Archives of Dermatology. Dermatologists knew the drug could increase levels of cholesterol, liver enzymes, and triglycerides that can raise the risk of heart disease, but they were surprised that in patients with normal lab tests *before* they started taking the drug 44% developed high levels of triglycerides and 31% developed high cholesterol levels and 11% developed abnormal liver tests.

Many patients' labs return to normal once off Accutane, but there are others who have been belittled for their inquiries suggesting the drug caused their diminishing health. Tom Shearer told his story on HoneyColony. com: "The root cause of my problems was impaired liver function, due to damage caused by the Accutane. That got the ball rolling and everything else followed as a result. It left me with very low bile production, resulting in chronic constipation and toxicity. The lack of bile also meant I wasn't able to digest fats properly, hence the vitamin D deficiency, as it is a fat-soluble vitamin." He's now working on healing his gut and his liver outside of a medical hospital where his issues began.

"Our figures show approximately four and one half million hospital admissions annually due to the adverse reactions to drugs. Further, the average hospital patient has as much as thirty percent chance, depending how long he is in, of doubling his stay due to adverse drug reactions." (Milton Silverman, M.D. Professor of Pharmacology, University of California)

Tom isn't the only one who's suffered the effects of the drug. Roaccutane, a brand name of the drug isotretinoin, is used by about 30,000 people in the UK each year. "Data from the MHRA's yellow card reporting scheme – a website for reporting adverse drug reactions – recorded 12 fatalities in 2019, 85 serious incidents and 19 non-serious ones. Since records began there have been 88 deaths," reports the Guardian.

In 2004, the Guardian reported that a promising medical student killed himself four weeks after being prescribed the acne drug. Jon Medland, in the last year of his medical degree committed suicide just four weeks after getting on the drug that sometimes exchanges beauty for life.

As concerns grew, the acne drug's pamphlet added, "some people have had thoughts about hurting themselves or ending their own lives, have tried to end their own lives, or have ended their lives. These people may not appear to be depressed."

Despite the number of suicides tied to it and successful court cases where its use has been found to have caused ulcerative colitis or Crohn's disease, Accutane is still being seen as a miracle drug for acne. (See Chapter Eight for more on Accutane.)

The users of the popular acne drug don't necessarily suffer from depression before getting on the pill. But many other teens and young adults are suffering with the invisible darkness while the Chemical Religion invites them into their false hope.

## Invisible Darkness

There's a tremendous amount of research alerting drug companies, doctors and consumers that there's a higher risk of severe adverse drug reactions including suicidal and aggressive behavior and overstimulation with mania and psychosis for children taking antidepressants. But what is a parent supposed to do when their teen is struggling with depression? It can be a helpless feeling when there doesn't seem to be any options.

We talked in depth about depression in Chapter Seven, but in this chapter, we want to address it again. Depression is something that so many young people battle and its worse now with social distancing and quarantines. Before the COVID nonsense, if our teens were isolating themselves, we would insist they get out and socialize, but today's world makes that difficult.

Did you know your teens became smokers? Oh, but you say they don't smoke. Well, 2020's quarantine debacle is the equivalent of smoking 15 cigarettes a day on health! Research shows that you can reduce your chances of cancer, type 2 diabetes, cardiovascular disease, and back pain, all with one simple lifestyle change: reduce the time you spend sitting. Sitting is more dangerous than smoking. It kills more people than HIV and is more treacherous than parachuting.

According to a CDC survey around the effects of the quarantine, our youth are at an increased risk of suicide with 25% of the young responding they had "seriously considered" suicide in the past month between March and June 2020. So many parents believe they're protecting their children by keeping them in when they may be endangering their mental health instead.

Robin Caruso of CareMore Health has research that suggests friendships reduce the risk of mortality or developing some diseases. They can even speed recovery in those who become sick. People need people. We *are* better together … without masks and without six feet separation. (See Chapter 12 for more facts on COVID-19).

Besides combatting loneliness with real connection, we can help our teens avoid or overcome the invisible darkness with movement. The average American teen spends seven hours a day looking at their screens. That's a lot of sitting!

Less than 3 in 10 high school students get consistent physical activity throughout the week according to the CDC's May 2018 report. Researchers at Duke University studied people suffering from depression for four months and found that with just 30 minutes of exercise three times a week that 60% of the participants overcame their depression without using anti-depressant meds.

Furthermore, typically active people who became inactive were 1.5 times as likely to become depressed compared to those who maintained an active lifestyle. This seems to indicate that an individual who would not normally face depression would now be susceptible in a quarantine environment.

While most fitness research efforts focus on the physical health benefits of exercise, there's a growing body of work demonstrating that exercise promotes wellness and mental health. It boosts self-confidence and helps prevent depression.

Movement, especially of the spine, is required for proper brain function. It's better than any smart pill for concentration and learning. It's a natural antidepressant for more stable emotions. And it enhances motor control which offers an edge to young athletes, and it keeps all organs functioning well for optimal overall health.

Roger Sperry, the recipient of the Nobel prize in 1986 for his work in brain research, stated that the importance of movement of the spine in relation to brain function could be equated to that of a windmill that generates electricity for a power plant. He also stated that the more structurally distorted we are, the less energy we have for metabolism, healing, thinking and functioning.

Depression isn't the only deadly consequence of a sedentary lifestyle. If you stand or move around during the day, you have a lower risk of early death than if you sit at a desk all day. Physical inactivity contributes to over three million preventable deaths worldwide each year, making it the fourth leading cause of death due to non-communicable diseases. Lifestyle sitting causes harm to the body in many ways and increases risk for:

- Metabolic syndrome
- Compression in the discs leading to premature degeneration
- Anxiety and depression - (see Chapter Seven for more on exercise and mental health)
- Cancer - (see Chapter Five for more on how exercise fights cancer)
- Heart disease - 147% higher risk of heart attack or stroke (60% of 15–19-year-olds had plaque building up in their coronary artery
- Diabetes - 112% higher risk of diabetes
- Varicose veins
- Deep vein thrombosis
- Adolescent obesity (According to the CDC it's tripled in the past 30 years.)

Movement that works up a sweat provides benefits that don't come with warning labels. Some of those are listed below:

- Kickstarts weight loss
- Promotes healthy weight
- Releases heavy metal toxins, urea, bisphenol-A and phthalates
- Improves blood flow, reducing blood pressure, and improving cognition

We were created with a major route to unload a lifetime of damaging, disease producing chemicals: SWEAT! Set the tone right away with your teens that exercise is not an option. It's a requirement! Exercise heals the body and the mind!

## Blowin' Smoke

Parents thought that tobacco had lost its allure for youth who grew up with anti-smoking marketing. So, when vape shops opened on every corner seemingly overnight many of us were completely naïve to not recognize that they were coming for our teens. Vaping quickly became an epidemic that often leads youth to take the next step into smoking pot. Somehow the FDA allowed it on the market bragging that it was a safe alternative to cigarettes. It wasn't long before the emergency rooms were filling up with kids who couldn't breathe, having one thing in common: vaping.

By early 2020 there had been 2,807 hospitalizations or deaths from vaping. EVALI is a new lung disease linked to this form of smoking. The name is an acronym that stands for e-cigarette or vaping product use-associated lung injury.

The symptoms EVALI are similar to those in other respiratory illnesses, like pneumonia and the seasonal flu virus. They include:

- Shortness of breath
- Cough
- Chest pain
- Fever and chills
- Diarrhea, nausea, and vomiting
- Tachycardia (rapid heartbeat)
- Tachypnea (rapid and shallow breathing)

Vaping is *not* safe. It increases your teens risk of developing lung disease by about 30% and causes "popcorn lung," the nickname for bronchiolitis obliterans. This irreversible condition damages and soon scars the lungs' smallest airways causing an uncomfortable cough and a scary feeling of shortness of breath.

E-liquid contains:

- Diacetyl: This food additive, used to deepen e-cigarette flavors, is known to damage small passageways in the lungs.

- Formaldehyde: This toxic chemical can cause lung disease and contribute to heart disease.

- Acrolein: Most often used as a weed killer, this chemical can also damage lungs.

- E-cigarettes contain a large dose of nicotine, a substance known to slow the development of brains in fetuses, children, and teens.

- Cancer-causing chemicals

- Heavy metals

- Volatile organic compounds (VOCs)

The American Heart Association indicates that vaping is not safe. They say the liquid that creates the vapor is dangerous to adults and children if they swallow it, inhale it or get it on their skin. They also warn vaping may normalize smoking again as it becomes more popular, especially among the youth. It's marketed almost like a candy store with alluring flavors. But, like candy lined with arsenic at Halloween, teens are unknowingly ingesting poison with each puff. When they were little, we use to check their candy for evidence it had been tampered with. Now that they're older we need to be just as diligent in checking the things they are consuming for their safety.

Being a parent to teens in today's highly influenced world of drugs is definitely challenging. So much has changed since we were kids facing drugs. We only had to *"just say 'no'"* to peers and drug dealers. But our kids are the target of marketing for drugs paid for by insurance benefits rather than with their saved-up lunch money. The susceptible aren't just the "troubled" kids anymore. The users are the studious, college bound and athletes working hard to be the best they can be. They're scared to fail. They're stressed out.

We can help our kids by reminding them what God says in Jeremiah 29:11NIV, "'For I know the plans I have for you,' declares the Lord, 'plans to prosper you and not to harm you, plans to give you hope and a future.'"

We need to teach our kids where the true source of happiness is found. It doesn't come from a pill bottle, a can or a vape. It comes from the love of God who holds their future in his hand, and he will not fail them. When they believe that, they'll be free from the lies and bondage of the Chemical Religion.

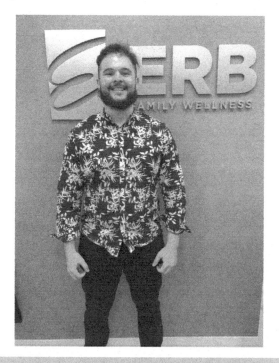

When I was a kid, I refused to eat anything but sugar and bread until I started getting teased for being chubby. My parents helped me to make some changes in my diet and showed me how to workout, but I was still driven by the harsh words. I got into bodybuilding, and I didn't care as much about being healthy as I did about being the strongest and the biggest.

I started drinking energy drinks to push myself, but eventually got into Adderall and steroids to increase my performance. I was taking 4-5 (100-125 milligrams) Adderall pills a day. I was also smoking pot, drinking, and vaping to numb the pain. I was on a dangerous road, and I didn't care what happened to me until I started seeing the effects. I had trouble breathing and developed all the signs of sleep apnea. I was going bald at 20 years old. I was angry all the time and anxious unless I was high.

I came to Erb Family Wellness after I was in a car accident. I had already stopped all my vices, but my hair was still thinning, and I had put on a lot of weight. The accident left me in so much pain I could barely make it through the examination without passing out. The pain was nauseating.

In two months' time I am now pain free and my hair has started growing back. Besides the spinal adjustments, I began eating healthier because I was feeling healthier under their care. I took their advice and started intermittent fasting. I haven't lost any weight yet, but I've been able to work out again and I am gaining my muscle back, but this time without steroids and high doses of caffeine. – Isaac Gates

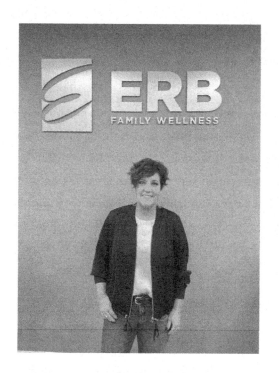

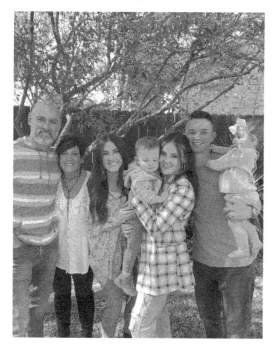

My family and I have been going to the Erbs for about 12 years. I had really high cholesterol when I started. It has gone down significantly since I have been under the care of Erb Family Wellness.

A couple years ago I was tired and not feeling well. I didn't really know what was going on with me, so I decided to do the metabolic test. My results were terrible. I was on a scary path towards disease.

Dr. Kimberly put me on a protocol that I followed to a T. She recommended specific vitamins and a strict diet plan. I also started exercising more. I began feeling a million times better and I lost 20 pounds! When I tested again it was evident that my gut was completely healed.

With more energy and better health, I was motivated four months ago to hire a personal trainer. I am working out five days a week and gaining a ton of muscle.

The Erbs have given us the knowledge we need about food, toxins, spinal care and exercise to better care for ourselves and for our grandchildren. We are all eating organic whole foods, grass-fed meats, and non-GMO products. I believe this lifestyle has also helped me get through the symptoms of menopause.

We are so grateful to the Erbs for speaking truth into our life about health. We are thankful to not be taking any medication. Even my grandbabies have been going to get adjusted. I believe this is why they have rarely been sick in their life. They have never had an ear infection. They have never taken medications or antibiotics. We didn't know these things when we were raising our kids, but we do now, and it has made a huge impact on the health of our family. – Kristie Tillman

# CHAPTER 11
# YOU'VE BEEN LIED TO!

"Moses was 120 years old when he died. His eyesight was sharp; he still walked with a spring in his step." Deuteronomy 34:7 The Message

The people in the Bible lived unbelievably long, spry lives. Sarah was considered beautiful enough to be taken into a king's harem when she was knocking at ninety's door. Moses was well into what we would now refer to as geriatric years when he climbed a mountain on his own to meet God. And Noah was about 500 years old when he started building a giant boat to save mankind. These people didn't have motorized wheelchairs to get them around. They didn't have Medicare. They didn't have regular checkups, hip replacements, heart bypasses or memory care facilities. How did they manage to live so long when in today's world forty-five is considered middle aged?

The leaders of old were respected for their age and their wisdom. "Gray hair is a crown of glory; it is gained in a righteous life" Proverbs 16:31 ESV. Age was respected in Bible times. The more mature weren't looked upon as weak. They were the patriarchs and matriarchs who were honored for the legacy they passed down to the next generation and beyond.

When I was a kid growing up, I didn't know anybody who had hip or knee replacements. Breast cancer wasn't an epidemic and people we knew lived into their nineties still mowing their own lawns and tending their gardens. We didn't have cell phones or annual exposure to radiation with painful breast exams smashing us down like pancakes. Our nutrition hadn't become wiped out the way it is now. Leaky gut, malabsorption and deficiencies all cause joints and bones to weaken. Back then we hunted, fished and gardened. Now people eat contaminated foods and trust in a healthcare system that seems to hasten their demise. Our forefathers and mothers are now hunched over and weak. Let's be clear it's not just age or genetics causing seasoned adults to suffer. It's the lifestyle choices in their youth that have caught up to them. It's believing the lie that they must slow down and move less with age. But it's not too late.

The mature adults of our modern society have been lied to for too long. Every year is a new opportunity to truly live and thrive. Age doesn't mean immobilization. It doesn't mean frailty. It doesn't mean irrelevancy.

## You've Been Lied to About Your Value

Elephants are known to travel like a family in packs, but poachers have been changing the natural structure of these innocent animals. The illegal hunters slay the largest males in the pack for their tusks. The fathers and grandfathers suffer and die leaving young males without role models. Now surprising reports are emerging of young, rogue elephants killing rhinoceros and attacking buses. It's out of character for the species to be so aggressive.

When the family structure designed by God becomes dismantled it's replaced with chaos. The roles of family are passed down through example, but if we don't protect and honor our parents and grandparents, we bring confusion to the younger generation about who they are and what they are to become. Right and wrong gets cloudy as true role models are replaced by culture's agenda pushed by media. It's an agenda meant to discredit the value of family and replace it with the influence of counterfeit puppets pushing worldly views and compliance.

As the elderly have been demoralized by the culture, we've been robbed of the wealth they have stored up in their experience. They feel they don't have anything worth sharing. They think young people don't want to listen. But without these seasoned humans to pass down their wisdom we are left to start over rather than being able to grab their baton and go further.

### Is Retirement a Disease or a Dream?

Retirement is the eternal vacation from a lifetime of work. Couples growing old together often spend their evenings dreaming of the day they can cash in on their retirement. They anticipate spending their golden years set free from the daily grind to do all the things they haven't been able to experience. But 25% of retirees soon realize it was all just a dream. Instead of traveling the world they are scraping by afraid they will run out of money before they run out of time.

There are retirement formulas that help seniors determine how much money they will need to retire, but Charles Schwab surveyed Americans and reported that most say they will need on average $1.7 million. The dream becomes a nightmare when adults reach 55 and are forced to work another ten years. But will the extra money be worth it?

Boeing produced a paper showing that employees who retire at 55 live to, on average, 83 years old. But those who retire at 65 only last, on average, another 18 months from the time of retirement. Lockheed Martin, Ford Motor Company and Bell Labs showed very similar numbers based on the number of months pension cheques were sent out before retirees died.

Waiting longer to retire while carrying fear that it still won't be enough adds stress. As we have discussed already, stress is toxic to the immune system. Prolonging their dream to retire for another decade must be a huge disappointment! The Bible affirms the impact emotions can have on health. "Hope differed makes the heart sick, but a longing fulfilled is a tree of life." Proverbs 13:12 NIV.

In nearly every chapter we have discussed how stress is poison, but can alleviating stress be a kind of fountain of youth?

One study compared the DNA of highly stressed mothers caring for a chronically ill child with women who were not dealing with such stress. Stress seemed to accelerate aging by about 9 to 17 additional years! Even perceived stress was associated with higher oxidative stress which in turn, accelerated aging. So, whether we are dealing with real issues such as when to retire or perceived issues that shift our focus from good, positive things for which we can be grateful, stress may be robbing us of precious years. If stress ages us, then maintaining a happy heart that hopes in God could prolong our days.

## What Happens When Veterans Become Isolated, Depressed and Trapped?

Among our matriarchs and patriarchs are those who risked their lives fighting for our freedom. Most of our veterans were just kids when they were exposed to the devastations of war. They were forced to take lives, to watch their peers suffer and die. They saw things on the battlefield that no human was meant to endure. And when the war was over, many carried all that they saw with them back home. The pain, the fear, the regret, the human conflict of it all was left undealt with and bore down on them creating a daily stress. They felt isolated by their experiences. Depression filled the spaces in between the war they remembered and the opportunity to live.

Many veterans don't want to rehash what they've been through and even if they did, they don't think anyone would understand. Often times, shame for the things they had to do in war haunts them, so they withdraw. Social Isolation among older adults is estimated to account for $6.7 billion in federal spending. The lack of good friends and family connection isn't just an invitation for depression. It has been associated with a 29% increase in risk of coronary heart disease and a 32% increased risk of stroke.

- Even chronic, sub-clinical mild depression may suppress an older person's immune system based on a study including participants in their early 70s and caring for someone with Alzheimer's.

- In a meta-analysis 300 studies on stress and health were reviewed and it found that people who are *older* or already sick are more prone to stress-related immune changes.

- Depression hurts the body's ability to fight infection, but does that mean pills are the answer for protecting our parents and grandparents from early death?

- 887,859 VA patients treated for depression were examined and found that completed suicide rates were twice the base rate following antidepressant use in VA clinical settings

Patient exposure to the SSRIs is currently estimated to exceed 85 million. That's scary when, like we explained in Chapter Seven, the dangers of antidepressants and SSRIs that block serotonin increase risk of suicide! Serotonin regulates the most important stimulator of calcium, therefore a Canadian study concluded that serotonin inhibitors double the risk of 'fragility' fracture from weakened bones.

There are all kinds of harmful side effects associated with these drugs, but elderly patients may be more vulnerable to the emergence of dyskinesia (abnormal or involuntary movement) after SSRI treatment. Dyskinesia is known by doctors to be a growing issue for patients who trust them not to prescribe anything harmful. But it has created an opportunity for Big Pharma to profit from producing another pill. Recently we saw a pharmaceutical commercial unashamedly advertising a pill specifically for SSRI patients who have developed dyskinesia. In fact, studies are showing a 100% chance of getting Parkinson's disease with SSRI use over time. If all these pills aren't the answer to helping our veterans, what is?

We've had many that come in and they are stuck in this diabolical VA system that says, "If you get better then you won't get paid for disability." Their monthly income is based upon *not* getting better. Several of our VA patients experienced this conundrum when they got well under our care. They had to decide between their health or paying their bills. It broke our hearts when they quit care because they were going to lose their income. They, like so many others, are slaves to the system. That is part of the Chemical Religion that even influences the government to keep it in power.

### You've Been Lied to About Your Healthcare

The mentality of health today is like walking on a tight rope without worry because health insurance is there to catch us should we fall. We don't take care of our health because we can land on the safety net comprised of "ever improving technologies" drugs, needles and surgeries. The net is a trap like a web we can't escape. When we fall into it, our life is slowly sucked out of us.

Medicare, which makes the rules for insurance companies, isn't interested in keeping people healthy. It states clearly in Section 2251.3 of its guidelines, "A treatment plan that seeks to prevent disease, promote health and prolong and enhance the quality of life; or therapy that is performed to maintain or prevent deterioration of a chronic condition is deemed NOT medically necessary" ... and therefore not covered." So, that explains why they don't cover chiropractic care.

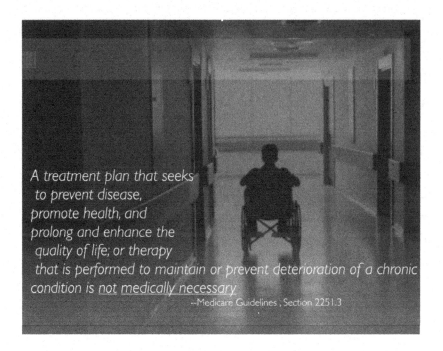

A treatment plan that seeks to prevent disease, promote health, and prolong and enhance the quality of life; or therapy that is performed to maintain or prevent deterioration of a chronic condition is *not* medically necessary
--Medicare Guidelines , Section 2251.3

A system that isn't meant to make people well makes them dependent. This is especially true for aged adults who are too often treated as though they are incompetent when they enter the hospital for care. They are degraded by nurses not wanting to deal with possible messes because they don't have time to walk the patient to the bathroom. Instead, the nurses put a diaper on people unnecessarily.

Older patients feel they've been treated like children in patronizing communication with their caregivers who are less patient, disrespectful and not as involved compared to how younger patients are treated. The physicians' attitudes seem to express less value for aging patients offering a pessimistic prognosis.

- One study found that nurses tend to assign a lower status to geriatric nursing compared to other practice areas.

- Another study indicated nursing trainees had a general lack of interest in working with older adults.

- A U.S. study found ageism to be a factor in under-treatment of patients with heart attacks. Older patients are less likely to receive standard diagnostic procedures and recommended treatments .

Medicare policies are not meant to incentivize hospitals or physicians to offer stellar treatment that could delay or prevent entry into a long-term care facility or hospice. Helping patients remain independent isn't their goal. Comprehensive outpatient geriatric care has shown to be beneficial as has part-time home care that assists frail patients in household duties. But Medicare does not reimburse for such liberating plans.

My grandmother ("GG") was in an assisted living home with Alzheimer's for about five years. It was a painful decision our family had to make, but my mom continued to be actively involved in her care. The staff kept her safe, but they couldn't fight with Medicare to get her the tools she needed to hold onto the last bit of mobility and self-sufficiency she had left. Her walker was being held together with duct tape. Grandmother's reclining chair that allowed her to get up and down without the help of a nurse was broken and her bed wasn't in good shape, either. Although these items were covered, we couldn't get Medicare to fix anything. Our family wasted so much time jumping through their hoops to no avail, until it was too late. When GG was put in hospice with only days to live, they were finally ready to answer our pleas, but what good were those things at that point! Furthermore, Medicare would not pay for her assisted living unless she agreed to let them drain all her cash and assets. How's that for a "safety net?"

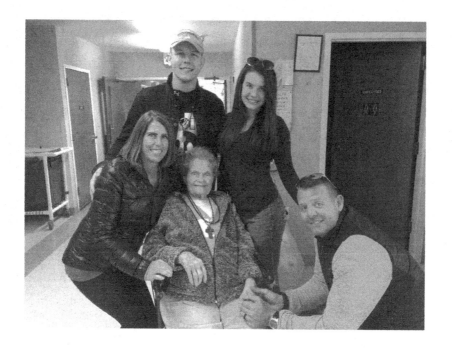

One thing we learned from tending to Grandma is that you can't expect caregivers and Medicare are going to take care of everything. Many elderly people will need a trusted mediator to ensure they get all that they need, or they will be neglected. They will be overlooked. They will be taken advantage of.

A 2015 study estimated that older Americans lose $36 billion each year from financial exploitation, criminal fraud and caregiver abuse. Plans that could protect patients from relying on untrustworthy caregivers while giving them freedom to be in their own home are unaffordable options for most.

Instead, Medicare doled out $18 billion to hospices in 2017. From 2012 through 2016, nearly all hospices that provided care to Medicare beneficiaries were surveyed.

- Over 80% had at least one deficiency.

- One-third had complaints filed against them.

- Over 300 hospices had at least one serious deficiency or at least one substantiated severe complaint in 2016 and were considered poor performers.

- What kind of deficiencies were discovered with these hospices?

- Neglecting background checks when hiring caregivers.

- Hiring caregivers without credential verification.

- Patient's rights complaints.

- Failure to monitor meds or communicate with the patients' M.D., resulting in wrong dosages or conflicting meds.

- Neglect causing sometimes *severe* consequences.

- Failure to track infections.

There were reports and stories of maggots in stomach feeding tubes, failure to clean wounds, resulting in gangrene requiring leg amputations, ignoring pelvic injuries from sexual assault and giving wrong treatment that put patients in the hospital.

Stories of hospice nurses giving high doses of morphine that kills patients saying, "It's just to take away the pain," are beginning to surface. Many of these patients spent their entire lives walking that tight rope, only to fall into its trap that eventually cost them their lives.

### They Steal Your Health Then They Take Your Memories

Years of mercury exposure from flu shots and teeth fillings accumulate on the brain along with all the chemicals people encounter daily eventually come to a head creating memory loss issues.

Alzheimer's and dementia are demoralizing diseases that reduce their victims to wearing diapers and an inability to even dress themselves. These disorders usually effect adults over 65 who have so much wisdom to pass down, but they can't remember anything anymore. It's a tragic loss for us all. Dementia cases have drastically increased. Data from the Global Burden of Diseases, Injuries and Risk Factors Study 2016 indicated the disease has grown by 117% between 1990 and 2016.

Another big business opportunity has been realized with the rising numbers. Memory care centers are popping up everywhere to accommodate adults who need 24-hour care protecting them from getting lost, forgetting to turn off the oven, or from endangering themselves in other ways. Many overwhelmed families come to accept that they are not equipped to properly care for their aging spouse or parent. They search out a memory care center or long-term care facility they hope they can trust, but the statistics are scary. When 2,000 nursing home residents were interviewed, 44% said they had been abused. Equally alarming, 95% said they had been neglected or seen another resident neglected.

By now you already know how we feel about vaccines, but let's talk about how the annual flu shot effects your parent's ability to remember you.

Metals like aluminum (used in cookware) and mercury (found in fish, tooth fillings and vaccines) are highly toxic. Thimerosal is a mercury-based preservative found in flu vaccines. This is what Hugh Fundenburg M.D., an immunologist who served for 20 years on the expert advisory panel in immunology for the WHO and has over 800 papers in peer reviewed journals had to say in his speech at the NVIC International Vaccine Conference, Arlington VA September 1997 about flu shots.

"If an individual has had five consecutive flu shots between 1970 – 1980 (the years of the study) his/her chance of developing Alzheimer's Disease is ten times greater than if they had one, two or no shots." Dr. Fundenburg is a noted researcher in Alzheimer's. His credentials prove his statement cannot be ignored as having come from an "anti-vaxxer."

Aluminum is another metal causing cognitive dysfunction. A study published in the *Journal of Alzheimer's Disease* on January 13, 2020, links exposure to aluminum with Alzheimer's. Researchers found significant amounts of aluminum content in brain tissue from donors with the disease. Stay away from drinking from cans and using aluminum pans and foil to cook your food.

Another study examined over 900 people without dementia and again after 3.6 years. They evaluated the group's muscle strength and the development of Alzheimer disease. The study determined that those who did not develop the disease had maintained more muscular strength in comparison with the ones who developed Alzheimer. That makes sense because physical activity has also been shown to protect people from developing Alzheimer's.

Once again, exercise emerges as a key factor in resisting disease. Making movement a continued priority as we grow older can be the difference between getting on the floor to play with our grandchildren or having them push us around in a wheelchair. The less we move the less we will be able to move: so stay active. Walk, dance, golf, enjoy life doing something rather than sitting if you want to avoid diseases like Alzheimer's.

We shared with you the truth about cholesterol and the dangers of taking medication to reduce it in Chapter Four. This includes memory loss. For the middle aged, symptoms and risks emerge such as erectile dysfunction and battling belly bulge. But those are just the warning signs of a bigger war you are facing in your golden years when you choose the way of the Chemical Religion.

The elderly have come to be automatically associated with joint pain, decreased mobility, memory loss, depression, heart disease and osteoporosis. We have been led to believe this is simply what we can expect with age. It makes growing old seem scary and we begin to feel powerless, but the truth is much suffering can be avoided by breaking free from the Chemical Religion. The sooner the better!

Statin drugs reduce cholesterol but may be one of the leading causes of what has become the picture of old age. Do these side effects sound familiar to the characterization?

- **Joint pain** (severe)

- **Decreased mobility**: Atrophy

- **Heart disease**: Heart failure

- **Depression**: Statins block the body from producing serotonin which opens the door to depression.

- **Osteoporosis**: Statins like Lipitor are proven to deplete the body of magnesium which is necessary for the body to utilize calcium. The mechanism of the drugs function assures eventual loss of bone density.

- **Memory loss**: Statin Induced Dementia

- Liver damage

- Neuropathy (numbness and tingling in extremities)

- Ligament rupture

These symptoms are literally describing the most common issues geriatric patients experience! Remember, in Chapter Four we warned you that statins block the body's ability to produce CoQ10, an important antioxidant needed to transfer energy from food to our cells? It helps to reduce inflammation and protects us from cancer and *aging*. It's also the primary building block for the cells in our brain and nervous system. Blocking it often causes Statin Induced Dementia, a term the medical doctors have come up with because of how common the issue has become.

Should we really be blocking the thing that protects injuries as they heal, especially with the bone density issues the elderly face? Statins increase the risk of osteoporosis and then reduce cholesterol, that protects injuries incurred from weakened bones.

When a young person falls, she will likely only suffer a bruise and maybe a skinned knee, but when an elderly person falls her entire health can become compromised. It's often the first opportunity for an osteoporosis diagnosis.

In one study of over 13,000 women experiencing hip fracture, it was discovered that post fracture death occurred in 23% of women just one year later. The numbers increased significantly with age. Nearly 32% of women 85 years and older died within a year of their hip fracture proving that taking risks with bone health should always be taken seriously when deciding upon treatment.

As with any other disease, pharmaceutical companies saw an opportunity to formulate a pill that makes them look like superheroes, but with side effects that only a villain would inflict. Their not-so-heroic osteoporosis solution should only be praised by the tooth fairy.

Fosamax (alendronate) is a drug prescribed by doctors to help patients develop denser bones. With everything we've talked about in this book it's not surprising that research shows it actually *causes* bones to weaken and crumble. Thigh bone breaks and osteonecrosis or jawbone death (the jawbone itself dies, resulting in tooth loss) has been reported. Women 60 and over taking the drug for two to five years are especially at risk. Fosamax has reports of side effects from 90,757 people. Among those, 1,595 people (1.76%) have tooth loss.

We had an older patient who was taking the drug and didn't understand why her teeth were falling out. We showed her that it was a side effect of Fosamax. Our patient wanted to get off it immediately, but her daughter insisted that her mom continue taking it.

We were seen as the bad guys for causing mom to question the M.D.s orders. It saddens us to see how intelligent people can remain convinced by the Chemical Religion cult even when the evidence is so strong against it.

A slew of other medicines that many older adults have been on for years have been linked to osteoporosis. How does that even make sense to give drugs with the potential to cause bone density loss to patients at risk for osteoporosis! Let's just say that taking one of these drugs listed below might not be enough to cause the deterioration of your bones. But think about how many of these are in yours or your parent's medicine cabinets.

- Heartburn drugs reduce acid production in the stomach thus reducing nutritional absorption. With less calcium uptake, more calcium is pulled from bones to replace it.

- Diuretics like Lasix (furosemide) cause the body to increase urination which increases calcium excretion from the kidneys taking with it nutrition. The body loses calcium, so it pulls calcium from bones to replace it.

- Blood thinners like Heparin used long term have been shown to reduce bone density. (It also causes thin skin and bruising, another issue we often associate with old age rather than with prescription use)

- Diabetes medications like Avandia and Actos have been shown to cause an increased risk of fracture when used four years or more.

- Acetaminophen users who took the drug regularly for at least three years showed an increased risk of fracture versus individuals who did not.

- Antacids decrease stomach acid contributing to chronic stomach acid production dysfunction issues which decreases nutrient digestions and absorption. Lack of proper nutrients means nutrition doesn't get to bones and thus bones weaken.

Life on the tight rope will eventually bring you crashing down into the treacherous net designed to ensnare you. Living a lifestyle without care for nutrition, avoiding exercise and exposing ourselves to toxins without caution is an accident waiting to happen. Putting our trust in a healthcare system that fills our medicine cabinets with pills that attack our body organ by organ is a dangerous path. The safety net is a deadly trap.

## What's All the Hysteria About?

Hysteria was the term used by physicians to describe neurotic conditions. The word was derived from the Greek word *hystera* meaning 'uterus' because the condition was originally a diagnosis given only to women. Apparently, physicians believed only women could have strong emotions or be "insane." The term, no doubt, perpetuated the culture's bias against them. At times it was used as an excuse not to take women seriously. For example, if a young lady chose not to marry, disagreed with her husband, or had a mind of her own to go against society's expectations in any way, she had a "wandering uterus" and needed to be *fixed*. We've come a long way, but still today women fight against this mentality that MDs once promoted. Though the term is no longer used as a psychological diagnosis, the root stuck when referring to the removal of the uterus.

Hysterectomies are one of the most common surgeries for women living in the United States. According to the CDC as many as 600,000 American women have hysterectomies each year. Whether for noncancerous tumors such as fibroids, heavy periods, endometriosis, a dropped uterus or for various cancers of the reproductive organs this procedure is just the beginning of a whole new set of problems. In some cases, as with endometriosis, a hysterectomy doesn't even diminish the symptoms. It's nothing but a physically, emotionally and financially draining experience.

Hysterectomy is *not* a cure for endometriosis according to the Office on Women's Health at the U.S. Department of Health and Human Services.

- There's a 15% probability of persistent pain even after the surgery.

- A 3-5% risk of worsening pain or new symptom development.

A hysterectomy should not be a first-line treatment. Alternatives are out there for about 90% of hysterectomies, according to Streicher in her book *The Essential Guide to Hysterectomy*. While we may not agree with many of the alternative treatment methods, the question remains, why would a doctor encourage such an extreme surgery when there are other options? Options that don't cut away at the core of what makes a woman a woman and leave them to deal with other issues such as:

- Postoperative depression

- Bladder dysfunction

- Pelvic pain from the scarring

- Inability to have a cervical orgasm

- Early menopause

- High blood pressure

- Obesity

- Heart disease

- Bone density loss

A study published in 2016 in the *Journal of Clinical Endocrinology & Metabolism (JCEM)* found that hysterectomy significantly increases the risk of developing thyroid cancer in postmenopausal women.

Women also experience other chronic pain after hysterectomy from organs that can shift after one is removed. Hip and back pain then radiates into their neck explained Heather Hirsch, MD an internist specializing in women's health at Brigham and Women's Hospital in Boston.

"Are we doing too many hysterectomies? I'd say the consensus among providers who perform them would be that there are probably too many performed right now," said Christopher Tarnay, MD, division chief of uro-gynecology and reconstructive pelvic surgery at UCLA.

- As many as one in five women who underwent the surgery for a benign condition may not have needed the procedure. For women under 40, that figure may be as many as two in five.

- About 90% of hysterectomies are done for reasons *unrelated* to cancer.

Why are so many of these surgeries being performed? Could greed have something to do with it? A Virginia OBGYN was convicted after he performed hysterectomies at his discretion for insurance fees. Do you think he's the only doctor who has performed hysterectomies for the money over finding the best solution for his patient? It happens more than what is reported because patients would have to realize the facts after they've already had the surgery. Then they would have to have the time and money to take their physician to court.

We were with friends in the hospital just after they lost their baby. We turned a wrong corner and stumbled upon a white board displaying a goals chart. The board promised a trip to Hawaii for all staff if goals were met. Several surgeries were listed such as gallbladder, colon, hysterectomy and more. In each surgery category there were hashtag marks indicating the number that had already been performed. Everyone was encouraged to upsell patients because, as much as people don't want to admit it, medicine is a business.

So many of these surgeons play God with people's bodies! "Let's remove this organ, you don't really need that organ and while we are in there, let's take this out too." I'm pretty sure God knew what he was doing when he created the human body, and my guess is that he didn't design us like a piece of IKEA furniture with extra parts that we don't need.

Hysterectomy surgeries are a lot like the recommended scheduled Cesarean. It's a conveniently scheduled, quick easy surgery, leading to more surgeries like bladder surgeries, breast cancer removal and fake hormones.

## You've Been Lied to About Hormones

Many women who have had hormone regulating organs removed will be the first to admit there were a lot of things they wish they had been told before making the decision. These ladies have usually gone through so many ups and downs trying to regain balance in their moods, regulate their body weight and regain their sex drive. Throughout the process relationships become strained from the emotional rollercoaster.

Oral hormone therapy should be entered into cautiously. Given the choice between healing your organs that can then regulate your hormones naturally or removing them, which do you think would be the best solution?

Patients facing this decision have been assured by their doctor that hormone replacement therapy (HRT) is identical to what your body produces, but rarely are they given any options outside of removal. Rarely are they told that HRT carries increased risks of stroke, blood clots like deep vein thrombosis and heart disease.

In Chapter Four we exposed how some medications effect our body's ability to produce hormones. In Chapter Eight we talked about toxins and xenoestrogens all contributing to Big Pharma's new money-making industry. Low-T and fem centers continue to grow in popularity. They offer hormone replacement therapy to regulate periods, potentially allowing for pregnancy, ease menopause symptoms and to boost testosterone for weight loss and muscle-building—at least that's what they preach.

Premarin is one option for estrogen replacement despite its questionable ethics for its treatment of animals. If women knew what they were putting in their mouths, we're not sure they'd be able to keep it down. Premarin is made of horse urine. Approximately 750,000 horses a year are impregnated and locked up in tiny stalls without room to sit comfortably, so as not to disturb the bags strapped to them. The horses aren't given much water, so the bags are filled with more concentrated urine increasing the potency for the pills. The mares are slaughtered and used for dog food once the pharmaceutical company no longer has use for these living beings.

In 2002, the Women's Health Initiative announced that it was ceasing a large clinical study on HRT medication due to findings that the drugs were increasing the risk of breast cancer by 26%, of blood clots by 100% and of stroke by 41%. The following other risks associated with HRT's have been discovered.

- Endometrial cancer (a type of uterine cancer)

- Gallbladder disease

- Heart attack

- Increased breast density (which some researchers believe may also increase the risk of developing breast cancer)

- Ovarian cancer

- Pulmonary embolism (blood clots lodged in the lungs that impede breathing and can be fatal without prompt treatment)

There are other options for regulating hormones and we can help. Getting your spine corrected, avoiding endocrine disrupting toxins and taking supplements to give your body what it needs to recover from all the environmental stresses should not be underestimated. We've even seen menopause reversed! One of our patients was a little upset when her periods returned after receiving regular adjustments. Subluxation can cause interference with thyroid and reproductive organs. If you have a choice to try an option that spares you from surgery, wouldn't you think that would be a good place to start?

Our top-of-the-line supplements can help too. One supplement can:

- Increase growth hormone and testosterone

- Decrease cortisol

- Continue fat burned after exercise for 36 hours

- Increase sensitivity to insulin

### You've Been Lied to About COVID

*Everybody's* been lied to about COVID and the jabs being marketed as vaccines. We'll talk more about that in Chapter 12. But our older citizens have been made to feel especially afraid. Yes, they are more at risk for mortality than their children, but the numbers are still in their favor. People 45-64 years old have a survival rate of **99.9294%** and those over 85 years old have a survival rate of **98.2499%.** So why are adults running out to take their chances with a vaccine that has not been properly tested? People taking the shot are pharma's lab rats.

The Office for National Statistics (ONS) data shows that weekly care home deaths tripled in the two weeks between January 8th and 22nd, 2021 after an increase in vaccinations among residents.

On January 16th, 2021, the British enclave of Gibraltar vaccinated the elderly with the Pfizer vaccine. The small territory populated by only 33,000 had the worst Covid-19 mortality in the world (2,761 per million) after the shots were administered. Prior to the vaccination there had only been nine COVID deaths up to December. In less than five months nearly one hundred people lost their lives.

A third of the residents died At Pemberley House in Basingstoke, a care home in England after Covid-19 vaccinations began. Prior to that the home of those mostly over 80 years old had been COVID free.

We have a patient in the medical field. He took me aside one day and in a hushed voice he said that 11 people had just died after being vaccinated in the nursing home where he worked. He said that nurses see it, physical therapists see it, but everyone is too afraid to speak up. They know they could lose their jobs or worse if they speak against what the Chemical Religion is willing to kill for.

The lie is that the risk of dying from the COVID virus is greater than the risk of dying from the shot. That's the message the Chemical Religion is broadcasting, but you have the power to change the station. You have the power to tune into the truth.

You've been lied to. You are *not* a burden to society. You are *not* senile or rigid. And being old-fashioned in morality and skills isn't anything to be ashamed of. Our society needs you to lead us back to some of those foundations. We've swayed off course and are calling evil good and good evil. You are our matriarchs and patriarchs to remind us from where we've come.

Moses, Abraham and others lived long, strong lives, but we have an even better covenant with God now through Jesus. We have the Holy Spirit to lead us into all truth. We have the blood of Jesus that gives the promise of salvation and healing. By His stripes we were healed. And in Chapter 13 we will share with you some tools that will allow you to work with God's design to keep your body functioning optimally like our forefathers.

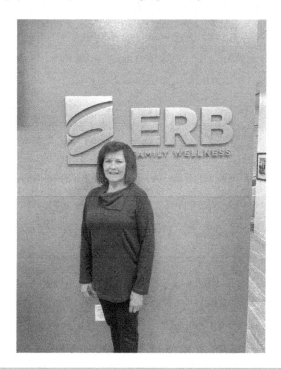

I was diagnosed with severe Sciatica in June of 2019. After my MD in Iowa did an MRI, he recommended that I get a cortisone shot to relieve the pain. The administering doctor said, "This shot is a band aide, you'll need to come back in three months for another one."

In October of 2019 I started coming to Erb Family Wellness and thought, "I don't want another shot. I'd rather just get well." I was pleased that Dr. Erb did X-rays before any adjustment, so she knew exactly what the problem was. Two years later I am still pain-free and still no shots are needed!

Getting everything aligned and keeping it aligned has made a world of difference in my general well-being. But most importantly I had an unexpected surprise after my adjustments. Dr. Erb was able improve the hearing in my deaf ear! I'm 74 years old and I had lost hearing in one ear when I was 5 years old. I wasn't aware of the hearing loss until I was failing second grade and discovered it was because I couldn't hear. Fast forward to 2019 after spinal adjustments my hearing began to return. I didn't realize it until my daughter and I were in a restaurant having lunch and from the booth behind us I could hear a man's voice in the ear that I had not used in years! My hearing is not yet 100% but it continues to improve as I get adjustments and become accustomed to using both ears rather than relying only on my 'good' ear.

I am so thankful that God sent me to the Erbs. They're more highly trained than any chiropractor I've ever known. The doctors and the entire staff are pleasant, kind, informative and encouraging as the team keeps my spine aligned and continue to teach me about good nutrition and general good health. – Denise Willhoit

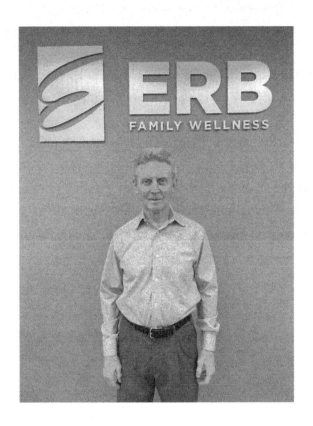

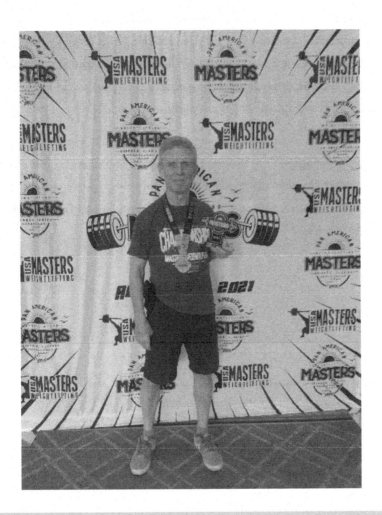

I have been going to Erb Family Wellness for about five years. I'm an athlete. I work out a *lot*. My principal focus is Olympic weightlifting. My main concern is to maintain health. I am in really good shape, but spinal care and removing subluxation is key to staying in good shape. When my previous chiropractor's office moved, I went looking for another quality chiropractor. After visiting the Erbs' office, I was convinced I had found one.

My years with Drs. David and Kimberly have been a continuation of a practice necessary to maintain optimal health. Since I have been under their care, I've won *two* world championships. I have won *three* national championships. I won *four* state championships and recently, this year, I won one Pan-America championship. The Pan-American is a competition within this global hemisphere from Alaska to the tip of South America. It's not quite as big as a world championship but it's a huge feat.

At 74 years old, most people my age are living a different life than I am. Some of the things I do in the gym are only appreciated by people who do gym work. I could not possibly do all of this if I were not executing my practices properly. Good chiropractic care is a part of the process.
– Bryant Stavely

# CHAPTER 12
# MASKING THE TRUTH

"For the time will come when they will not endure sound doctrine, but according to their own desires, because they have itching ears, they will heap up for themselves teachers; and they will turn their ears away from the truth and be turned aside to fables. But you be watchful in all things, endure afflictions, do the work of an evangelist, fulfill your ministry." 2 Timothy 4:3-5 NKJ

In 2020 the world blindly accepted propaganda that would disempower the people, weaken economies, and increase the suicide and domestic violence rates, all while fueling an agenda meant to make Big Pharma and its affiliates more power and money.

We gave away our rights without a fight in exchange for protection from a virus that was rumored to have been intentionally spread. We gave up our right to assemble and embraced social distancing; we gave up jobs and businesses in exchange for government assistance if we promised to not leave our homes; we wore masks because if we refused, we would be harassed by strangers (in fact, shaming and bullying anyone not complying was encouraged).

Day and night people religiously watched the news and were brainwashed by the propaganda. Anyone who dared to question the message was scorned as selfish and uncaring. The brainwashed became indignant when their beliefs were disproved by real evidence. The slogans were everywhere! The message came across fast and clear as if the signs had already been designed and printed. It all seemed so strategic.

- #AllAloneTogether
- We Are in This Together
- #StayHome
- Please Remember to Wash Your Hands
- You Are the True Heroes
- Staying Apart is the Best Way to Stay Connected

- **New Normal**
- We'll Be Stronger on the Other Side
- #SocialDistancing
- Good Hygiene is in Your Hands
- We will Heal Our Land
- During These Uncertain Times

In 2015 Dr. Peter Daszak, president of EcoHealth Alliance, an organization that conducts research and outreach programs on global health, conservation, and international development said, "We need to increase public understanding of the need for medical countermeasures, such as a pan-coronavirus vaccine. A key driver is the media, and the economics will follow that hype. We need to use that hype to our advantage to get to the real issues. *Investors will respond if they see profit at the end of the process.*" (Emphasis added) Suggesting a need for a pan-coronavirus vaccine five years before there's a coronavirus pandemic? Using the media to drive hype for their economic advantage? What we have experienced is starting to seem more calculated than we would like to believe.

The term "New Normal" isn't actually new and seems to be a part of the strategy. It was first introduced on January 6th, 2004, at a conference called *SARS and Bioterrorism: Bioterrorism and emerging infectious diseases, anti-microbials and immune modulators.* The pharmaceutical company Merck suggested the term as a way to get people to accept a universal pan-influenza, pan-coronavirus vaccine. It was adopted by the WHO and the Global Preparedness Monitoring Board, on which the Chinese Director of the Centers for Disease Control, Bill Gates, Dr. Elias of the Gates Foundation and Anthony Fauci "happened" to sit together. The WHO, Fauci and, of course, Bill Gates quickly emerged as heroes. The world looked to them for their salvation. Gates would give directions and the rest would immediately echo. But were we just sheep being led to the slaughter?

## How About Those Numbers?

The CDC was a kind of false prophet. The people looked to the federal agency (with its $11.1 billion budget) for hope yet it refused to tell the truth that could set them free from fear. Its website indicates that for a pandemic to be declared there must be a 7% death rate from the disease.

The WHO had already changed their definition of pandemic as if in preparation for what was to come. Prior to the swine flu "pandemic" of 2009, the term was defined as, "An influenza pandemic occurs when a new influenza virus appears against which the human population has no immunity, resulting in several, simultaneous epidemics worldwide with *enormous numbers of deaths and illness.*" (Emphasis added) If the change had not been made to replace "deaths" with, *"a worldwide epidemic of a disease,"* neither the swine flu nor the COVID virus currently receiving so much attention would have been considered a pandemic.

Covid has not proven to be the cause of "enormous numbers of death." The most recent numbers, refused to be shared by the media, would allow the world to go back to the *old* normal. No masks, no online school, no vaccines, and none of this government deciding whose livelihood is essential.

These percentages prove how *non*-essential it was for people to lose jobs, homes, businesses, their mental health and overall wellbeing to avoid spreading what isn't much more than a yearly flu. The recovery rate by age is as follows:

- 0-14 years old survival is 99.9998%

- 14-44 years old survival is 99.9931%

- 45-64 years old survival is 99.9294%

- Over 85 years old survival is 98.2499%

Dr. Kelly Victory posted some facts that were since removed from the web for not matching the media's script.

- 20% of common colds are caused by corona virus, Covid-19 is a mild disease

- 85% of people who contract it have little if any symptoms

- 10% or so become ill with flu like symptoms and need to seek medical care

- Only a small number of those require hospitalization

Every year flu deaths range from 60-90 thousand. Every life matters, but death is a part of life on earth. To put into perspective why so many of us were not convinced that such measures were needed, Covid deaths accounted for about 142,755 deaths out of 3,952,273 total cases reported when all this was heating up. About 3,809,518 people recovered. There were more deaths in 2019 before the pandemic than there were in 2020.

If we're going to shut down for Covid, then we might as well shut the world down for the yearly flu or common colds. All this evidence has gone unnoticed, ignored or is getting deleted. Fear and misinformation have spread faster than the virus. By July 2020, announcements were being made that schools would not reopen for the first three weeks.

Dr. Mercola (and others), following true numbers and science, have explained that children are safe from Covid. Just look at the numbers above! Furthermore, you're not going to kill grandma by exposing her to your kids who have spent the day among peers. There's a low risk from exposure from children who have the Covid virus in their nose or mouth. They harbor less than 25% of the viral load found in adults, which is likely why they don't become sick.

The numbers have been manipulated from the beginning. The CDC website that had become a kind of Covid bible wasn't forthcoming that pneumonia and influenza deaths were included in the COVID-19 numbers making the "pandemic", quarantining, mask-wearing and school closures all seem a bit unnecessary. But everyone was drinking their Kool-Aid so to speak.

Professor John Ioannidis referred to the so-called pandemic as "a fiasco in the making." He wrote about the lack of accurate data and the tendency to ignore information that would make all the drastic measures sound ridiculous. He stated, "If we had not known about a new virus out there, and had not checked individuals with PCR tests, the number of total deaths due to "influenza-like illness" would not seem unusual this year. At most, we might have casually noted that the flu this season seems to be a bit worse than average."

Unfortunately, his advice was ignored and instead Neil Ferguson of Imperial College of London had predictions that better suited the agenda. He professed that 500,000 people in the UK and two million in the U.S. would die unless drastic measures were taken. Had everyone forgotten how wrong his predictions were on other diseases? In their book _Corona False Alarm? Facts and Figures_ Dr. Karina Reiss and Dr. Sucharit Bhakdi share some of Neil Ferguson's past predictions.

In previous years he prophesied 136,000 mad cow disease deaths, 200 million avian flu deaths and 65,000 swine flu deaths. When these diseases finished running their courses, they only accounted for a few *hundred* deaths each. This false prophet's recommendations were the science that was believed over the facts. And that's the kind of science that the media, CDC, the WHO, Fauci and Bill Gates (the guy without any medical credentials) have used to force worldwide pandemic protocols.

Most people didn't notice the subtle change in terms made by the CDC to manipulate numbers. "Probable cases" was replaced with the term "confirmed cases" on their website. That meant that if you went to the hospital with any one of a long list of symptoms you were likely diagnosed a probable case and included in the COVID-19 numbers. Obviously, that made the number of cases look more intimidating, but the forces behind the agenda were hungry for more numbers. Fear thrives on lies.

Senator Scott Jensen says that hospital administrators may pressure physicians to cite all diagnoses including "probable" COVID-19 on discharge papers and death certificates. Texas, for instance, had to remove 3,484 "COVID" cases from their count, announced Steve Edgar of Fox 4 News in Dallas/Ft. Worth. He further stated that the San Antonio Health Department was reporting "probable" cases for people never tested as confirmed cases. We wonder how many other less conservative states had unchallenged numbers.

Maybe scarier than the deceptive numbers were the lists made from those testing positive. You may remember they called it "contact tracing," when phone calls were received by responsible citizens demanding they come in to get tested. In 2020, if you had been listed as having come in contact with someone who tested positive for the virus, you could be subjected to a painful test against your will. A swab would be forced through your nose, nearly reaching your brain to determine if you had been infected. If found guilty (your "crime" being a positive test) you might be put on house arrest.

The fearful people who were watching the news couldn't understand why those of us who were better informed saw these things as complete violations of our rights. We were scared too, but for very different reasons. We were scared the vaccination that was being tested in Africa would be forced upon us, along with the deadly side effects it had inflicted on the people there. We were scared for the future of our children who were receiving lesser educations and suffering greater control from a government that was lying to them. We were scared for our country's ability to recover and thrive economically again lest it fall prey to socialism. And we were scared for the ways that friends and family were so viciously turning on each other.

The number of cases may have seemed to be growing, but did that mean the number of deaths were rising?

In May of 2020 a concealed document surfaced on the METI website (the German Ministry of Economy, Trade, and Industry) that exposed the real reason the numbers and facts weren't making sense with the government's actions to enforce shutdowns. The high number of Covid cases were being reported intentionally versus the low number of deaths because those would "sound too trivial," the document stated. Planned, premeditated fearmongering was exposed in this page of their website, which was conceived in mid-March 2020. When numbers were declining, governments would give more tests to increase the number of positive tests. This would drive people to be more afraid of the virus. But these tricks were not being reported. Not in Germany, not in the UK and not in the U.S.

In March 2020 Professor Walter Riccardi, adviser to the Italian Ministry of Health, went on record with the Telegraph that 88% of the Italian "coronavirus deaths" had not been due to the virus. Furthermore, examination of the facts proved that almost 96% of COVID-19 virus deaths had preexisting conditions and the average age of those who died was over 80 years old.

The Times of London reported on April 15, 2020, that England and Wales had experienced a record number of deaths in a single week. Was it from corona? Nope! Only half of those extra numbers may possibly be due to the virus. It was from people in need of care who were avoiding the hospital for fear they might expose themselves to COVID. Others died who were in need of surgeries that had to be indefinitely postponed while the hospital focused on COVID patients.

Beds were being held for coronavirus patients who never came, while patients in need of surgeries and other non-COVID related care were suffering at home. Many died because 30 million elective surgeries were canceled or postponed worldwide in the first 12 weeks of the pandemic. In Germany and in the U.S., hospitals were empty, and thousands of U.S. physicians were put on administrative leave because routine outpatient visits dropped so significantly. It seems that what was considered *essential*, saving hospital beds so doctors could save the lives of COVID patients, made other patients' care *non*-essential. Who decided which lives were worth saving and which ones were nonessential?

At least 42% of U.S. coronavirus deaths are from .6% of the population, the elderly. Initial numbers were high because those living in long-term care facilities were forced to share space with the infected. "They [long term care facilities] don't have a right to object. That is the rule, and that is the regulation," New York Mayor Cuomo stated, "And they have to comply with it."

New York was the center of our epidemic. As of May 2020, more than half of our nations COVID-19 deaths occurred in this liberal state with its policy ordering long-term care facilities to admit COVID-infected patients discharged from hospitals. New Jersey, Massachusetts and California were also hit particularly hard by the virus. They too ordered facilities housing the elderly to admit recovering coronavirus patients. The policy meant to free up hospital beds to make room for sicker patients was a death sentence for those most at risk. Why were hospitals preferring COVID patients over others?

Fudging patient numbers is a financial win for hospitals and further fuels fear. USA TODAY reported that Medicare gives $5,000 for, say, pneumonia but if the discharge papers or the death certificate says "COVID-19 pneumonia" the hospital gets $13,000. Documents that say COVID-19 pneumonia *with* ventilator is their jackpot. Hospitals gets $39,000 when they get to ventilate a patient even if it's just a probable case.

Dr. Deborah Birx of the American Coronavirus Task Force also admitted that the U.S. national Covid death count is actually much lower than what was being reported. Unlike other countries, the deaths reported are of people who died "with" COVID-19 rather than those who died "from" COVID-19. That would mean that death certificates are being falsified. Families who have lost people they love are being used to further spread fear because when asked, "How did he die" they repeat what they are told: "Covid."

When I (David) worked at the busiest emergency room in the U.S. I was responsible for taking the deceased to the morgue and generating the paperwork including the death certificate. I was the first point of contact for ambulances carrying people including those who had died in transit. I am very familiar with death certificates.

The initial line indicating cause of death in a death certificate is where the actual cause of death is stated. There are several lines following that indicate possible contributing factors. If the cause of death is lung cancer, one of the indicated "due to" lines might list smoking. Smoking is not the cause of death but if the deceased had not smoked, he may not have developed lung cancer for instance.

The rules have changed since Covid. Here is what's happening to boost hospital income and fuel fear of death by coronavirus. If the cause of death is heart failure or pneumonia, but there is a "due to" line or even an "other significant conditions" line that lists Covid, the death is included in the fearmongering numbers.

One man in Florida died in a motorcycle crash. Because he had recently been COVID-positive he was certified as a COVID death. Another publicly reported instance of this kind of fraud occurred in Colorado with two gunshot victims. Both of the deceased had tested positive weeks before and therefore added to the COVID deaths numbers.

Hospitals weren't the only ones exaggerating the numbers. At least one high official was fighting for the truth. President Trump sought to hold accountable reports and reporters. The administration confirmed what many knew was happening. The CDC had been inflating the COVID-19 numbers so grossly that the administration had to strip them of control of the viruses' data, reported White House correspondent Emerald Robinson. The numbers were redirected through the White House first. Trump also stopped funding the WHO in January 2020 and threatened to cut off money permanently until they can prove they are no longer corruptly influenced by Communist China after they lied to our country about human-to-human transmission of COVID-19.

The lies around Covid have been dulling the senses of many. They have been like a fog that kept intelligent people from seeing the truth. The fallacies lulled them into a slumber from pursuing what common sense suggests. Even when deceptions have been exposed the masses have remained blinded from the truth. The CDC admitted they screwed up COVID-19 infection counts, which misled the public. They clarified that the number of people truly infected is much lower than what was originally reported. The truth was uttered but so many could not hear. They remain asleep in the lies that seem to comfort them.

## Social Distancing

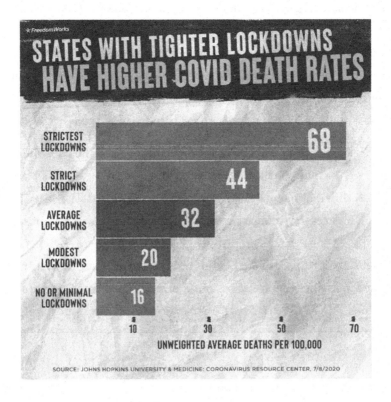

We are unapologetically huggers. No one enters our offices without receiving at least one big loving squeeze. None of this halfhearted side hug business is extended in our offices: we go the distance! We believe hugs heal, and there are studies that back up what we practice. Hugging has been found to:

- Reduce anxiety and stress

- Increase oxytocin, which is associated with happiness. (Levels rise when we hug, touch, or sit close to someone else.)

- Boost heart health

The isolated are twice as likely to die prematurely, making it comparable to smoking and alcohol consumption for risk of death. Loneliness and social isolation can be as damaging to health as smoking 15 cigarettes a day.

Socially isolated individuals have a 30% higher risk of dying in the next seven years, especially among the middle-aged, according to an analysis pooled data from 70 studies and 3.4 million people. It increases the risk of heart disease by 29% and stroke by 32%. Stats like these prove that "All Alone Together" isn't a good plan for staying well. God said, "It is not good that man be alone." We were created for togetherness.

The effects of isolation and social distancing start early. The hormone levels of babies and children who have been deprived of physical contact are significantly different than of those who have been cuddled. They have higher levels of the stress hormone called cortisol. Young adults who were socially isolated as children have significantly poorer health. There are several possible reasons for this. Isolated children have been found to lead increasingly sedentary lives and refrain from exercise. They may smoke and drink more, possibly as a form of self-medication. They also tend to grow up more stressed.

Our poor babies are going to need lots of hugs if they are to recover from the travesty inflicted upon them when their schools were shut down! Kids missed out on events they dreamed of their whole lives like prom and homecoming. They missed out on things they worked so hard for like graduation ceremonies and sporting events.

The best thing we could have done for our youth and for the overall health of the world would have been to allow kids to be exposed on their campuses. Herd immunity may have been attainable through those most resilient to Covid. As we stated above, kids 0-14 years of age only have a .0002% risk of not recovering. Most kids exposed have mild symptoms if any at all. It's even unusual that they would pass Covid on to adults, so teachers, parents and grandparents are not at a greater risk when kids assemble. Instead, our kids received lesser educations from stressed teachers scrambling to create classrooms for online learning. And for what?

The CDC confirmed a .2% deathrate for COVID-19 and for that, as we write amongst growing depressive economic numbers, the U.S. has suffered unimaginable loss. We have:

- Added nearly $6 trillion to national debt
- Laid-off or furloughed 50 million workers
- Placed 60 million on food stamps
- Gone from 3.5% to 14.7% unemployment
- Crippled the petroleum industry
- Ruined the tourism industry
- Bankrupted the service industry
- Destroyed food industries and supply chains
- Threatened, fined and arrested church leaders
- Exacerbated mental health problems skyrocketing RX drugs
- Shut down schools and colleges
- Given unbridled power to unelected officials
- Increased suicides
- Delayed surgeries and treatments for profound illnesses
- Infringed upon countless important civil liberties
- 46% of small businesses have closed and will never open again.
- Placed 300 million Americans on house arrest

Written by JD Hall / Courtesy of Tara Thralls

Social distancing isn't even an established healthcare concept. It's never been scientifically proven. Quarantine is a viable concept, but the sick are the ones isolated not the whole world. Keeping the healthy isolated from one another isn't necessary. In fact, a New York study showed that 66%

of all COVID hospitalizations have been among people who wore masks, washed their hands, practiced the six feet rule and stayed home. Social distancing and following all the protocols have not protected the people. Instead, it has brought unimaginable harm.

The UN estimated 500 million people could become impoverished worldwide from the shutdowns, but no one seems to care. So much for the pre-Covid mission to solve world hunger. The mission now is to prevent worldwide exposure to a virus with a .2% or lower deathrate. How does that make sense?

David Beasley, Head of the UN World Food Program warned the UN Security Council that the shutdowns would cause a "hunger pandemic of biblical proportions." He explained, "It is expected that lockdowns and economic recessions will lead to a drastic loss of income among the working poor. On top of this, financial aid from overseas will decrease, which will hit countries like Haiti, Nepal and Somalia, just to name a few. Loss of revenue from tourism will doom countries like Ethiopia since it represents 47% of national income." Like many others before and after, his reasonable voice has been ignored and millions have suffered for it.

All the government-imposed shutdowns have America facing recession. Hundreds of thousands of businesses closed permanently in New York state alone from the restrictions. Retirement savings have been destroyed, leaving many wondering how they will recover. How will they survive? Covid has been a true killer but not for the reasons reported. Like in the days of the Great Depression, people have been killing themselves because they can't imagine recovering from their financial losses. The Australian government estimated a rise in suicides of up to 50%, 10 times higher than the number of COVID deaths. I wonder if Covid was listed on the death certificates so they could also be included in the fraudulent numbers.

An ABC-TV affiliate in California reported that doctors at John Muir Medical Center tell them they have seen more deaths by suicide than

COVID-19 during the quarantine. "The numbers are unprecedented," said Dr. Michael deBoisblanc, referring to the spike in suicides. "We've never seen numbers like this in such a short period of time," he added, "I mean, we've seen a year's worth of suicide attempts in the last four weeks."

There has been a large group of people who didn't look to suicide as their answer. Instead, they turned to drugs and alcohol. Even before COVID, 88,000 Americans were dying from alcohol related illnesses every year. But the dark joke of quarantine became the skyrocketing sales of alcohol. What wasn't so funny were the recovering who returned to their deadly comforts during the quarantine. Others who had not abused alcohol before found themselves pouring another glass past what they knew as responsible consumption. One alcohol home delivery company increased their sales by 350% while bars were still on lockdown.

It's no longer unusual for us to go into a consult with a patient who confesses to drinking a bottle or more of wine a day, or who is hiding in their closet drinking their dinner.

A *Wall Street Journal* report said quarantine has caused increased drug use for anxiety and insomnia. Prescriptions for anti-anxiety medications such as Klonopin and Ativan, rose 10.2% in the U.S. from March 2019 to March 2020 according to data from health-research firm IQVIA. Prescriptions for antidepressants, including Prozac and Lexapro, rose 9.2% in the same period. Increased use means increased dependency. When quarantine lifted, many were still being held hostage by their addictions.

Whether from the substance abuse, the stress associated with not being considered "essential," or from shear fear, domestic violence cases went through the roof. Imagine those kids who were already facing such terrors after school, but now there was no school. And now their abuser was home all day, too. Who would come to their rescue? Where could the victims go to get away until mom or dad calmed down?

Johannes-Wilhelm Rörig, the German government's commissioner for abuse, urgently cautioned that there was strong evidence that Wuhan's domestic violence tripled during their initial quarantine. He also stated that Italy and Spain had "alarming numbers." Violence in the home became a new epidemic ignored by those who also ignored the science that said, "Let's go back to the way things were."

A new normal comes with abuse, poverty, revoked freedoms, and all kinds of things that are definitely not normal. Is this really the best Americans can hope for? It seems an injustice to our founding fathers if we let this happen to our nation. Benjamin Franklin once said: "Those who would give up essential liberty, to purchase a little temporary safety, deserve neither liberty nor safety."

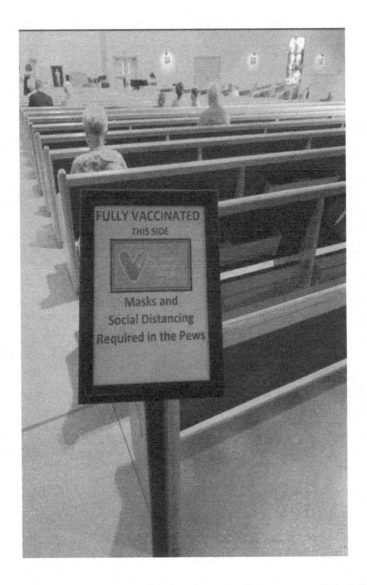

We've been giving our patients healing hugs for their spine and their hearts for over twenty years. We hate seeing how social distancing is starving people from the essential human touch. So many of our patients were forbidden to say goodbye to grandparents before they died. One of our dearest friends has suffered knowing her dad died alone. No one was allowed in to hold his hand or to comfort him in his last hours. These people did not have Covid. They died from noncontagious causes, but even if coronavirus was a factor, it is inhumane to prevent family from being there for each other.

### Silenced By the Masks

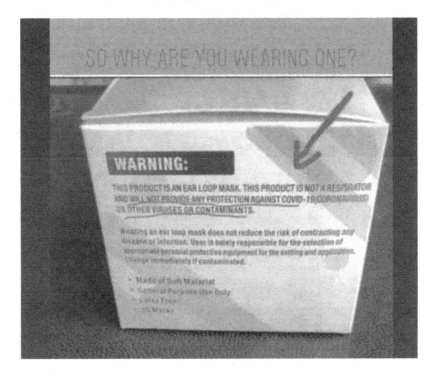

There's much to be said about masks. Granted, most of it doesn't make any sense. Yet the world has been walking around looking like they're wearing diapers on their faces. It's almost like the governments are trying to see if we'll let them strip us of our dignity by making us look more and more crazy.

The masses complied with the mask mandate because they just wanted free from house arrest! But then the CDC took it a step further and suggested everyone wear two masks or better yet, they suggested "placing a sleeve made of sheer nylon hosiery material around the neck and pulling it up over a cloth or medical procedure mask." (Because that doesn't look at all ridiculous.)

We remember when those wearing masks were the suspicious ones. If someone walked up to you wearing a mask you knew you might be about to get shot. Now if you walk up to someone *without* a mask people are afraid you're going to kill them with your cooties.

Even though a lot has been said against wearing masks, people keep holding tight to them the way a child drags around a security blanket. Dirty, sticky fingers touching the material, touching food, touching the mouth, touching friends and family, spreading the love along with the yuck.

Who hasn't reused their mask that's moist from the warmth of our breath and saliva then tucked it into a dark pocket creating the perfect environment for bacteria to thrive? Then who hasn't reached into that same pocket and reapplied the mask on the way into the grocery store where we will use our hands to push a cart, touch produce, or the keypad at checkout? The surgical masks may be able to catch saliva droplets before they shoot out at other shoppers, but not from the viruses in the droplets that are a thousand times smaller than the pore size of the mask. Nor from the viruses that are all over our hands from the contaminated mask and from itching our face or adjusting our mask.

Here is a collection of surprising or conflicting statements made by government or medical officials:

- The U.S. Surgeon General warned, "You can increase your risk of getting it [Covid-19] by wearing a mask if you are not a health care provider," He added, "Folks who don't know how to wear them properly tend to touch their faces a lot and actually can increase the spread of coronavirus."

- In March 2020 the CDC recommend that people who are well should not wear a face mask (including respirators) to protect themselves from respiratory diseases, including COVID 19.

- The WHO put this statement out: "However, there is currently no evidence that wearing a mask (whether medical or other types) by healthy persons in the wider community setting, including universal community masking, can prevent them from infection with respiratory viruses, including COVID-19."

- The Journal of American Medical Association said, "Face masks should not be worn by healthy individuals to protect themselves from acquiring respiratory infection because there is no evidence to suggest that face masks worn by healthy individuals are effective in preventing people from becoming ill."

- The Annals of Internal Medicine posted, "In conclusion, both surgical and cotton masks seem to be ineffective in preventing the dissemination of SARS–CoV-2 from the coughs of patients with COVID-19 to the environment and external mask surface."

- Even though Dr. Fauci himself originally stated, "Right now in the U.S., people should not be walking around with masks . . . It might make people feel a little bit better, it might even block a droplet, but it's not providing the perfect protection that people think that it is. And often there are unintended consequences: people keep fiddling with the masks and they keep touching their face."

- Mask packaging warns of their uselessness in protecting wearers from Covid-19 and all the other statements against them. We still saw people driving around *alone* in their cars wearing masks because of the false information being shared by the media.

Even though the experts made it very clear that they were unnecessary there was still mask frenzy. It didn't help matters when the CDC and others who seemed caught in the Chemical Religion's agenda changed their story and began pushing the facial nuisances. Their stories that contradicted themselves didn't make sense. Why should we be forced to wear masks for fear of spreading a virus that was less deadly than the yearly flu?

"While this is a contagious virus and many people can be infected, to-date person-years of life lost from COVID-19 worldwide is probably in the range of 100- to 1000-fold less than the person-years of life lost from influenza in 1918" said John P.A. Ioannidis, MD, DSc Professor of Medicine, of Epidemiology and Population Health, and (by courtesy) of Biomedical Data Science, and of Statistics and Co-Director, Meta-Research Innovation Center at Stanford (METRICS), Stanford University, Stanford, CA said May 6, 2020.

Facts like these have not been reported. Fear of noncompliance was preached so that most dared not question the real risks of the measures being taken. Never mind that the Occupational Safety and Health Administration regulations state that an atmosphere of less than 19.5% oxygen can cause death. But when we wear a mask, we are exhaling only about 16% oxygen along with poisonous carbon dioxide. That means we are inhaling less oxygen than what is already considered deadly. How much worse it must be for those double masking!

Never mind that masks force us to breathe carbon dioxide endangering compliers with poisoning. The combination of low oxygen and carbon dioxide toxicity has equaled hypercapnia for many whether they realize it or not. You may have experienced some of these symptoms and didn't even know ripping off your mask would cure you.

# HYPERCAPNIA

*Can be caused by rebreathing your own exhaled C02 by wearing a mask continually*

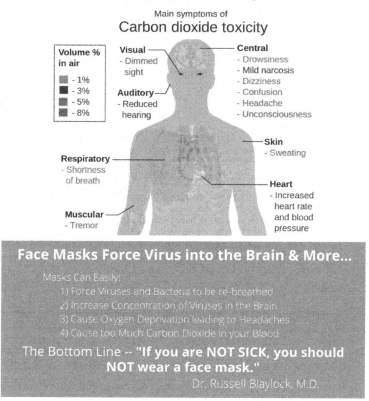

Main symptoms of
## Carbon dioxide toxicity

| Volume % in air |
| --- |
| - 1% |
| - 3% |
| - 5% |
| - 8% |

**Visual**
- Dimmed sight

**Auditory**
- Reduced hearing

**Central**
- Drowsiness
- Mild narcosis
- Dizziness
- Confusion
- Headache
- Unconsciousness

**Skin**
- Sweating

**Heart**
- Increased heart rate and blood pressure

**Respiratory**
- Shortness of breath

**Muscular**
- Tremor

**Face Masks Force Virus into the Brain & More...**

Masks Can Easily:
1) Force Viruses and Bacteria to be re-breathed
2) Increase Concentration of Viruses in the Brain
3) Cause Oxygen Deprivation leading to Headaches
4) Cause too Much Carbon Dioxide in your Blood

The Bottom Line -- **"If you are NOT SICK, you should NOT wear a face mask."**

Dr. Russell Blaylock, M.D.

People were suffering from headaches and other symptoms from lack of oxygen. Hypercapnia or carbon dioxide toxicity occurs when our lungs are forced to inhale carbon dioxide, dust, bacteria and viruses that are exhaled. Wearing a mask continually will affect our vision, central nervous system, hearing, skin, heart, respiratory system and muscles. They force viruses to be re-inhaled and increase concentration of virus into the brain. The exhaled viruses can even be forced into the part of the brain connected to memory through nasal passages called the olfactory. Our health has been compromised for fear we might catch a virus that had supposedly become a pandemic.

We discuss the health benefits of increased oxygen intake through exercise and how it prevents and fights cancer in Chapter Five, but it's important here to understand that decreased oxygen decreases immunity. Wearing a mask to keep us from getting sick is making us more likely to get sick.

Medical writer Dr. Russell Blaylock wrote in April 2020 on the heightened risks of face masks, "We know that the people who have the worst reactions to the coronavirus have the highest concentration of the virus early on." It stands to reason that mask wearers will have a higher concentration of the virus since they will have re-inhaled the virus and their masks will likely be filled with thriving virus. It also stands to reason that, since Covid-19 is a respiratory virus that the best thing we can do to prevent getting terribly ill from it is to protect and strengthen our lungs … by breathing in fresh air, mask-free. But never mind that, instead we have been forced to stay inside and to mask up.

Never mind the impact for those who have had to wear masks all day. Some dentists have noticed a new condition they call "mask mouth."

Mask mouth symptoms include:

- Sour breath
- Receding gums
- A dry mouth
- Tooth decay

Keeping your mouth closed and under wraps or breathing through your mouth more than your nose can dry it out. As it becomes dry of saliva that's necessary for optimal oral care, your breath starts to smell and your teeth suffer.

Never mind the truth. Don't look for it. Don't listen to it. Don't believe it. And certainly, don't speak it! That is the message of the Chemical Religion, and masks are the current the symbol of our compliance. It's really easy for those of us not under their spell to be identified with our refusal to wear them. We have suffered bullying of all kinds for daring to disagree.

In Texas, Deirdre Hairston was threatened with handcuffs and arrest during Holy Mass for not wearing a mask. She was six months pregnant and holding her one year old baby. Her head pastor turned her in while an usher taunted her, basically calling for her to be stoned.

Our rebellion is not just about the discomfort of wearing a muzzle or that they are physically harmful. Masks are an invasion of rights and a symbol of how we are being silenced, stripped of our identities and our voice. In the words of Martin Luther King Jr. "Freedom is never voluntarily given by the oppressor; It must be demanded by the oppressed."

Medical doctors and nurses, virologists, chiropractors and anyone else with information that speaks against the rehearsed media script have been silenced by the media and by those who control technology.

In July 2021 Donald Trump filed suit against Big Tech for their blatant censorship of anyone who is speaking against the sinister agenda. As we write this book, citations are being removed by Google, YouTube, Facebook and Twitter. Big Tech and the owners of each of these have removed truthful information. We were even put in "Facebook jail" for talking about the benefits of Vitamin D but we weren't alone in the discrimination. There were at least *200,000* Facebook users deleted who claimed adverse reactions to the Covid-19 vaccine.

Leaders in the field of vaccines are also being censored. During a July 6, 2021 interview Dr. Robert Malone, mRNA vaccine inventor and bioethicist, spoke out about his social media being banished. "Maybe some say I am the expert. But when you block my ability to communicate, let alone all the others that have contacted me saying, 'Hey, I can't even say the things that you've been saying, so speak for me,' now they don't even have me as a voice. That's profoundly disturbing. We can't get to scientific truth if we can't discuss things."

*Nobel Prize winner in Physics, Richard Feynman said, "I'd rather have questions that can't be answered than answers that can't be questioned."*

The year 2020 is the year of *pey* (a Hebrew word for "utterance"). It was the year to speak, and we were silenced through censorship of social media and by masking.

## Hand Sanitizer Insanity

People went crazy when the word "pandemic" started being broadcast. Even the quarantine couldn't stop the fearful from rushing stores and emptying them of anything labeled "antibacterial." From cleaning products to hand sanitizer, shelves were ravaged of these products that were supposedly banned years ago. Now people are dousing themselves and their children with them.

Triclosan was banned in 2016 and was supposed to be removed from the shelves by 2017, but as recently as July 25th, 2021, we were shopping and curiously read through ingredients to find that it was still listed. Triclosan has been linked to some serious conditions such as:

- Abnormal endocrine system/thyroid hormone signaling

- Weakening of immune system

- Increased chance of developing allergies, asthma and eczema in children exposed early

- Uncontrolled cell growth

- Developmental and reproductive toxicity

- Liver damage

- Increased risk of liver cancer

People are exchanging their potential of contracting a virus for contracting cancer. The Environmental Protection Agency warns that when triclosan reacts with sunlight it becomes a potent carcinogen. Also, when combined with our chlorinated tap water, it forms chloroform, yet another cancer agent. Virus or cancer: which would you rather take your chances of overcoming? We've already explained the numbers to you. COVID isn't the death sentence that the media has made it out to be, but cancer is another story. According to a 2013 publication in the *Journal of Gastroenterology & Hepatology*, studies show that by taking antibiotics or over cleaning our homes affects the microbiome or gut health in a way that can contribute to seasonal or food allergies, asthma, obesity, digestive issues like IBS and autoimmune disorders. Triclosan stores itself in cells and has been found in breast milk and blood. It threatens immune health, fertility and pregnancy. An abundance of studies have proven that higher levels of this antibiotic chemical is associated with seasonal allergies, hay fever and blocked nose.

Considering that Covid-19 is a virus that affects the ability to breathe, it seems that all this bathing in hand sanitizer might be a bad idea especially when the American Medical Association says that there is no evidence that suggests that using antibacterial soap works any more effectively than regular soap. A comprehensive study at the University of Michigan showed that it isn't any better at preventing both gastrointestinal and *respiratory* illnesses.

"Consumers may think antibacterial washes are more effective at preventing the spread of germs, but we have no scientific evidence that they are any better than plain soap and water" explained Janet Woodcock, MD, director of the FDA's Center for Drug Evaluation and Research.

Do we think that the more we sanitize the less bacteria we will have until one happy day all the world will be germ-free because we did our part to save mankind from its destruction? It would be nice if there was some sort of nuclear bomb we could employ to take out disease once for all, but if you understand bacteria then you will understand why trying to kill it makes it more dangerous.

If germs are the enemy, then using antibacterial products is only making our enemy stronger. Bacteria mutates with the resistance of such things as triclosan, which contributes to what's called, "bacterial resistance." These little germs are smart! Their defense against attacks is to become stronger and stronger. With each squirt of hand sanitizer, or wipe of a Clorox cloth containing antibacterial ingredients we are getting closer to programming a germ to be so strong even antibiotics won't be able to save us from its affects within our body.

Another problem with antibacterial products is that it kills microbiome organisms. Most microbiome organisms living in and on us are helpful to digest food, protect against infection and maintain reproductive health. All this sanitizing is only contributing to the problems people are trying to avoid.

## COVID Testing

PCR testing is to Covid what bullets are to a gun. A gun without bullets can still be used as a weapon in the way a baseball bat can, but it rarely kills anyone. The coronavirus could not have accomplished all the shutdowns, the forced masks, and welcoming of an unapproved vaccine without Covid-19 cases. Suddenly the annual flu went away and all that was left were coronavirus diagnoses confirmed by a flawed system of testing.

The creator of the PCR (which has been used as the main source for COVID-19 testing) calls PCR useless for indicating accurate results. Dr. Kary B. Mullis, Nobel Prize winner for his invention of PCR said, "The PCR: if you do it well, you can find almost anything in anybody." He explains, "The tests were never designed to tell you if you are sick." The leaflets that come with the tests warn that they are not approved for diagnostic purposes. So why are we using them?

Dr. Michael Yeadon, former VP and Chief Science officer of Pfizer, published his expert opinions September 2020. He said "we're basing our government policy, our economic policy and the policy of restricting fundamental rights presumably on completely wrong data and assumptions about the corona virus. If it weren't for the test results that are constantly reported in the media, the pandemic would be over because nothing really happened." Nothing *really* happened because the problem wasn't deaths and massive sickness. The problem was a failed testing system.

To understand what's wrong with PCR testing you need to understand how it works. A swab is taken from the patient and ran through the PCR, which is able to double the size of invisible molecules. With each cycle anything can be doubled again and again until it becomes visible. This sounds pretty cool until you realize that with enough cycles the virus has been found in everything from goats to chicken wings. The inventor had already warned everyone. If you can amplify it, you can detect it.

Dr. Anthony Fauci also admitted on a TWIV broadcast that a cycle threshold over 35 is going to be detecting "dead nucleotides", not a living virus. Not that we put any stock in Dr. Fauci, but even the guys who are calling the shots can't seem to get their science right.

The truth is that anything over 35 cycles is considered completely unreliable and scientifically unjustified. Already 70-90% of positive PCR test results generated using 35 or higher cycle thresholds (CT) are false positives. But when people start to feel safe and numbers are needed to keep control, tests have been set to as high as 45 cycles. This obviously produces many false positives. Some of what is being detected are pieces of debris, which may signal nothing more than a common cold in the past.

It's been interesting how the standard number of cycles have decreased as people started running to get vaccinated. The decreased false positives seemed to indicate that the jabs were working. Fewer COVID cases were reported until those who were hesitating needed more convincing. Cycles were increased which increased the Covid numbers sending a few more to get the shot out of fear.

Even now as this story evolves, pressure is rising. Those of us who remain jab free are resisting as a matter of life or death. We choose life over travel. We choose our health over career if necessary. Come what may, we know that this isn't going away just because we take a shot. There will be more shots to come and each one will inflict more disaster upon the recipients while blaming the resistance for the deaths of many.

Mark my words. I (Kimberly) did a talk called Tired or Toxic in January **2016** and predicted what is currently happening. You can find the talk on our YouTube ErbFamilyWellness. I said, "They are trying to come to Texas to take our rights away so we can't choose. By 2020 the agenda is to get all adults vaccinated. That's the agenda. In the name of Jesus that's not happening, but that's the agenda. And what that means is they won't give you a passport, a driver's license, a ticket to fly on an airplane unless they can see that you've had all your vaccines. The Bible says, 'Money answers all things.' So, you just follow the money on that. It's not about our welfare, it's about the money. So, we've got to be really vocal about this to make sure this doesn't happen to our children and to us."

There's currently a class action lawsuit for the crimes against humanity involving PCR tests for the part they played in the devastation from lockdowns. 1,000 lawyers have come together with 10,000 doctors in a lawsuit to see justice served for what they are calling the "2$^{nd}$ Nuremburg Tribunal." PCR testing fueled the corona fraud that technocrats such as the CDC, the WHO and the Davos Group for their crimes against humanity. The experimental vaccine violates all 10 Nuremburg Codes.

The PCR test has loaded the gun with fear's bullets. More tests mean more bullets. With less than a .2% risk of death, COVID is basically shooting blanks. Stop loading the gun. Stop the fear and **resist.**

## Are Ventilators Heroes or Villains?

Even though medical students are taught that ventilators should be used only in severe cases and for as little time as possible, these devises were praised as the heroes of COVID patients. Countries were stocking up on them and doctors were being instructed to use them in ICU beds. Hospitals were even rewarded with an extra $39,000 when they used a ventilator on a COVID patient. But are they safe?

The idea that infected patients on a ventilator would protect hospital staff from catching the virus actually put patients and staff further at risk. Ventilated patients require more care and cannot be ignored or risk of hospital-related injuries and infections occur such as what our friend and patient experienced in the testimony his ex-wife provided in this chapter. The medical profession wasn't naive to the fact that ventilators come with a high risk of lung infection or pneumonia, but for whatever reason they were putting ventilators on patients who didn't need them and were leaving them on longer than what many patients were able to recover from.

Are ventilators the heroes they were made out to be? Professor Gerhard Laier-Groeneveld from the lung clinic in Neustadt, Germany warned that intubation should never be used. Instead, he cured his COVID patients with non-invasive oxygen masks. He didn't lose a single patient.

Professor Thomas Voshaar, Chair of the Association of Pneumology Clinics, after losing the only patient he put on a ventilator (and the only patient that died) said that the high death rates in other countries, "should be reason enough to question this strategy of early intubation." There were a lot of doctors who saw near 100% recovery rates from their patients without using such extreme measures. These MDs cared more about saving lives than the $39,000 incentive. They are the true heroes.

The Chemical Religion is always preaching "early detection," except in the case of positive coronavirus cases. Before COVID patients could always count on leaving the doctor's office with some sort of medication. But with the exception of a few good doctors, COVID patients have been sent away empty-handed without so much as an antibiotic. Why are so many doctors not even trying?

Since President Trump stopped U.S. funding the WHO is heavily funded and influenced by the Bill & Melinda Gates Foundation. As we have seen, Bill Gates has spearheaded all things corona. Most nations adopted the health protocols from the WHO, including the decision not to treat the sick at the onset of the first symptoms. Instead, nations have waited for patients' symptoms to worsen turning into acute bilateral pneumonia to be hospitalized and ventilated.

We have a reflex-like tendency to reject new knowledge. It's referred to as the "Semmelweis Reflex" when we refuse to consider information that contradicts our belief system. Semmelweis Reflex has been deadly at times in medicine when evidence begins to conflict with what has become traditional medicine. This is also true when it comes to COVID. Many MDs have been led to believe that it's untreatable, therefore when their patients test positive, they don't consider what other doctors are saying about treatments.

Dr. Peter McCullough is a cardiologist and professor of medicine at the Texas A&M University Health Sciences Center. During a recent Texas state Senate Health and Human Services Committee hearing he said that data shows early treatment could have prevented up to 85% (425,000) of COVID-19 deaths.

Dr. Thomas Borody is a gastroenterologist and infectious disease specialist in Sydney, Australia who has discovered cures for ulcers and Crohn's. According to Dr. Borody, the tri-combination of ivermectin, doxycycline, and zinc is a near complete cure for the outpatient treatment of COVID. Dr. Borody says, "it is just hard to believe how simple it is to cure the Corona virus."

Dr. Borody isn't the only doctor who has been able to treat patients effectively with safe and proven methods. Doctors all over the world are saying the same thing with nearly a 100% cure for the virus. They may not have made as much money as the doctors who wait to ventilate, but these more ethical practices should not be ignored. Instead, patients with weakened immune systems return home with no knowledge of the supplements that have helped so many recover quickly. It isn't explained to them how to avoid the virus turning to pneumonia or other lung issues. Many have returned to the hospital in serious condition because their doctor didn't do anything before it was too late.

Once in the hospital, families aren't allowed to be by the side of their sick loved one. They can't offer input into the care being urged or decided upon without consent. Yes, many have died on ventilators who, if they had been given the option, would have chosen another method for their recovery. Even those most at risk might have chosen to spend their last hours awake holding the hands of their family. Way to go, ventilators!

### Injecting Us with Lies

While many doctors were seeing outstanding recovery rates with treatments that have been proven safe for years, the government and the media succeeded in silencing their good news while insisting that the only way the world could survive the coronavirus was if a vaccine was produced.

This wasn't just about dollar signs. Pharmaceutical companies were a part of a more sinister plan. Taking advantage of the people's fear and the government's urgency to start stabbing the population, the two powers struck a deal. The pharmaceutical companies demanded total immunity for damages including deaths that may arise from their latest potion. No wonder they were so insistent given their history.

These four vaccine producers Glaxo, Sanofi, Pfizer and Merck have in the last decade paid $35 *billion dollars* in criminal penalties, damages and fines for lying to doctors, for defrauding science, for falsifying science and for killing hundreds of thousands of Americans knowing their drugs to be harmful. Their hottest new product is no exception, except that they are protected from lawsuits.

The Public Readiness and Emergency Preparedness Act (**PREP Act**) frees pharmaceutical companies from taking any responsibility for the effects of their shots. Anyone taking the Covid jab will be asked to sign a release form along with their informed consent. But there's been no information to be obtained by the not-really-tested vaccine. Many people have unknowingly signed their lives away.

*"Science is too delicate for market forces to govern. It turns scientists into salesman" - Bret Weinstein*

"We want people vaccinated and we don't want to expose pharmaceutical companies to the kind of liability that they would otherwise have," said Brent Johnson, a partner with Holland & Hart, who defends corporate clients. "That's the price we're willing to pay to get rid of this horrible coronavirus problem." But what about the price the innocent will pay in their bodies for trusting these criminals?

The Covid-19 mRNA vaccine is exempt from what is common practice. If data from other studies suggest that the vaccine may affect physiological safety, then further studies must be done to determine toxicity. Responsible protocols continue to be ignored even with growing adverse reactions including deaths:

- No studies were done to see how the shot interacts with other meds.

- No toxicity studies were performed on a single dose.

- No toxicokinetic studies were done to see how these chemicals react once they are inside of a human.

- No genotoxicity studies were done to see if these chemicals damage DNA.

- No carcinogenic studies were performed to see if the injection would cause cancer.

- No studies were done on how it effects prenatal and postnatal development in moms and newborns.

- No studies have been done to see what happens when couples get the injection and on any subsequent children they may have.

This *thing* being promoted like it's the salvation of humanity is not even a vaccine! Vaccines cause an immune response to produce antibodies from a specific virus that has been injected through the shot. The Covid-19 vaccine is an experimental injection that causes the body to produce spike proteins, *not* antibodies. No one knows how long the production of spike proteins will last or even whether your body will ever shut off.

There is a big difference between vaccines and the mRNA injections. Our cells contain DNA that tells them what to do. The shots that are being misrepresented as vaccines contain mRNA which basically overrides our DNA. It reprograms our God-given design that will now take orders from a synthetic counterfeit made in a lab. Don't be fooled. These so-called vaccines do not prevent infection. They distract and disable our natural immune response.

For the unvaccinated, Natural Killer cells (NK) in our immune system kill the virus. Antibodies come after to clean up what's left. This is how populated areas overcome such viruses. Until October 2020 this process was called herd immunity. Seemingly in preparation for the big vaccine push, the WHO changed the scientific definition. It ignored the natural process of immunity and praised immunity through vaccination instead.

After protests from medical professionals the WHO had to change the definition again. On December 31, 2020, they included natural infection but continued their emphasis on vaccine-acquired immunity.

The science indicates that getting the virus, especially when we are young is our best defense long term. There was a SARS CoV-2 around 2004 that was very similar to the SARS of today. The blood of those who had been exposed show that those who were infected still have immunity. This is great news for all who have had this new strain. It indicates that not only are those who contracted either disease immune for at least 17 years, but maybe even for life. Boosters are not needed when you have contracted the virus naturally. Trust your body. God designed you to overcome.

### Neither Safe nor Effective

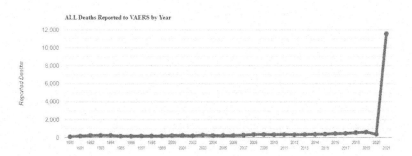

Through July 16, 2021

Reported Deaths post COVID Vaccine: Total 11,405

ALL Deaths Reported to VAERS by Year

Despite how the powerful have tried to hide it from the public, the "vaccines" are made mostly from graphene oxide. Graphene oxide (GO) is also the main ingredient in hydrogel liquid, which is the AI template used in

Elon Musk's and Bill Gates' research creating an interface in humans and the Internet. It's a material often referred to by chemists as a bioweapon. In taking the shot one must trust that the only code change they are injecting is one to stop the virus, even though the possibility of further hacking is a risk.

Pharmaceutical companies have been eagerly working on a plan to get graphene oxide on the market before the public was ever aware of Covid-19. Prior to the Chemical Religion's big break in acquiring an Emergency Use Authorization for their vaccine the key ingredient could not be approved. Graphene oxide had failed two trials on animals. The substance initially seemed promising in beating cancer but ultimately killed **all** animals injected. It was found to be toxic to healthy cells and caused Antibody-Dependent Enhancement (ADE). This is a huge problem when you realize that Graphene oxide is being used in a "vaccine" supposedly meant to protect us from a deadly virus. We will need a properly functioning immune system rather than one that is destroying itself from Antibody-Dependent Enhancement (ADE) if we are to fight it off along with variants and all future viruses that come our way.

Karen Kingston, former biotechnology analyst and marketing specialist with Pfizer, is a whistleblower who went on record confirming what was proven in a study out of Spain and China. The vaccine is 99% graphene oxide. The patented product lists this deadly ingredient as a "trade secret" and is therefore hidden from public knowledge. GO comes with a long list of reasons to be concerned:

- GO fibers are in plastic masks.
- GO fibers are on PCR test swabs.
- Is in all Covid-19 vaccines.
- Creates thromboses.
- Causes blood clots.

- Disrupts the immune system.

- Can trigger a cytokine storm.

- GO toxicity can instigate pneumonia.

- Creates a metallic taste in the mouth.

- Causes inflammation of the mucous membranes.

- Produces a loss in the sense of taste and smell.

- Is magnetic (especially at the injection site.)

- Blocks detoxification in the body by blocking glutathione.

- May be activated by 5G frequencies.

- Passes thru the blood-brain barrier.

The FDA's Vaccines and Related Biological Products Advisory Committee got together to discuss if the vaccine should be approved as an experimental injection for emergency use. The Acting Chair Arnold Monto, who has received money from Pfizer as recently as December 2018, presided over the committee. He shut down some targeted questions stating, "We aren't going to worry about adaptive innate immune responses right now." In an effort during the FDA virtual meeting to clear Covid-19 vaccines for the U.S. he said, "I think we want to stay away from discussions about immune response and other things that could be taken offline." It seems as though evidence against the shots was present but being hushed.

Other concerning studies from the past have been ignored. A 2002 study on Sars-Cov spike proteins showed they cause inflammation, immunopathology, and impede Angiotensin 2 expression (a narrowing of blood vessels that can cause kidney failure). The concern doesn't seem to be for the health of the public as much as for the Chemical Religion's offering plate.

Pfizer enjoyed the big break when the FDA allowed for their vaccine to be included in the Emergency Use Authorization. It became Pfizer's top seller, but the side effects have increased sales of some of their other top products.

The shot brought in $7.84 billion from direct sales and revenue split with its partner, Germany's BioNTech. That's nearly half the company's revenue. Pfizer expects 2021 to reach $33.5 billion for the 2.1 billion doses it's contracted to provide by year end.

Eliquis is Pfizer's drug for preventing blood clots and strokes. It just so happens that the sales jumped 16% to $1.48 billion in the quarter since the distribution of Pfizer's COVID jab, which has been found to increase risk of blood clots and stroke. Numbers don't lie. Follow the money, find the truth.

Once released, people flocked to the vaccine stations like sheep to the slaughter. Incentives and sweepstakes enticed the hesitant. These shots were even given for free *en mass* as governments pushed to be among the world's most-jabbed. It's been excruciating to watch the naïve getting in line to be injected with what has offered no sincere promises and has caused such devastation.

The promise was that the vaccine would eliminate masks and social distancing. That hasn't happened. The promise was that the vaccine would protect people from getting coronavirus. The vaccinated are still getting it and are passing it to others. The promise was that everything will go back to normal has been a dangling carrot since the "two weeks to flatten the curve." Now the Chemical Religion is promising that if more people take their shot we will finally be released from its punishments. But eyes are beginning to open to what's really at stake.

Remember, only about one percentage of adverse reactions are reported. Within the first 30 days that these injections began there were:

- 4,000 adverse events
- 3,100 anaphylactic shock
- 5,000 neurological cases

There's a long list of potential side effects that come with the vaccine that has still not been approved by the FDA as of September 2021. There are already tens of thousands of vaccine injuries being reported to the Vaccine Adverse Reporting Event System (VAERS).

- New, deadlier variants emerging from these leaky vaccinations (COVID shots)
- Menstrual irregularities
- Reproductive dysfunction
- 62% of vaccinated show micro-clotting systemically that can cause stroke
- Cardiomegaly (heart enlargement) from thickening blood
- Antibody Dependent Enhancement (ADE), which may also cause enhanced respiratory disease and acute lung injury

Thicker blood is causing more work for the heart, which in turn causes hearts to progressively enlarge. This is how and why not just youth, but all vaccinated people are seeing extremely high rates of heart issues. An enlarged heart can cause blood clots, which can block blood flow and lead to a heart attack, stroke or pulmonary embolism (clot in the lung). It may even lead to heart failure.

Autopsies performed on the jabbed are showing spike proteins accumulating in organs. This may lead to:

- Infertility when found in female organs.
- Leukemia related to bone marrow accumulation.
- Dementia/cognitive decline from the accumulation on the brain.

No product on the market has inflicted this much damage without being pulled immediately. Those of us refusing to subject ourselves to such risks are being treated like the Jews were just before Nazi's started apprehending them. The culture turned on the Jews based on hate propaganda derived from lies. If fearful people are told that the unvaccinated are dangerous carriers and transmitters of a deadly virus and that they are selfishly refusing to consider the safety of others, then fear will justify whatever treatment is forced upon them. It's only been 75 years since the Nazi's were defeated. Could history already be repeating itself?

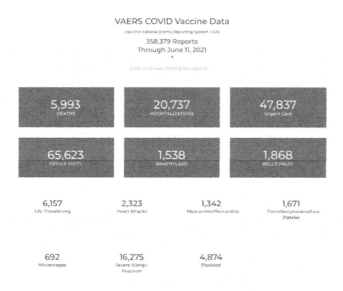

VAERS COVID Vaccine Data
(Vaccine Adverse Events Reporting System, USA)
358,379 Reports
Through June 11, 2021

For more than 20 years we have been bringing hope to the medically hopeless. We have been helping people break free from pharmaceutical drugs, pain and disease. Our offices have been a place of hope and healing. But for the first time we are facing some uncertainty as we learn more about these so-called vaccines. The virus doesn't scare us. But what top virologists are saying about these jabs has us on our knees before God more than ever. Jesus is the Great Physician who has been cleaning up man's messes since the beginning of time. Many people have ignorantly taken the shots, even people for which we care deeply. That's why it's hard to share this truth, but even now we are actively pursuing God for a way to reverse what has been done in ignorance. God is bigger than any virus and He is bigger than this injection.

It's important to understand that we aren't getting our facts from some radical antivaxxer/conspiracy theorist with no credentials. World-renowned vaccine creators and other experts in the field are putting their entire careers on the line because they are so concerned about stopping this genocide.

DVM has a resume that, just to name a few, includes:

- Senior Program Officer, Global Health, Vaccine Discovery for the Bill & Melinda Foundation
- Head of Adjuvant Technologies and Alternative Deliveries, R&D at GSK Biologicals
- New Biotech Vaccine Development and QC-QA Manager at GSK Biologicals
- Senior Project Leader 'Adolescent Vaccine Projects' at GSK Biologicals
- GAVI Program Manager

He has spent his life as a leader in the science of vaccines. To get people in his field to stand up and protect humankind against this vaccine, Vanden Bossche publicized a letter on his LinkedIn page March 2021 to beckon the WHO and all stakeholders to stand up against the distribution of the vaccine and declare what he calls, "The SINGLE MOST IMPORTANT PUBLIC HEALTH EMERGENCY OF INTERNATIONAL CONCERN."

The dedicated virologist and vaccine expert says that scientific evidence is being ignored and a "global catastrophe without equal" will likely be the outcome of the mass vaccinations. He explains that humanity is in danger of **viral immune** escape. The UK, Israel and U.S. vaccinated millions of people in just a few weeks. He predicted that though they may be boasting declining Covid-19 cases, they will start to suffer a steep incline of Covid-19 cases in the weeks to come. He was right!

Vanden Bossche, soon after his publicized letter, warned that we are already very close to vaccine resistance, explaining the vaccine will cause recipients to lose their ability to fight off any variants of any kind. The mRNA vaccines cause you to lose your innate immune response. "IT'S ALL GONE. Your innate immunity has been completely bypassed. This is pure science. We will pay a huge price using this [vaccine] during a pandemic."

Luc Montagnier was quoted in a post on RAiR Foundation USA. He said, "It is the vaccination that is causing the variants. You see it in each country, it's the same: the curve of vaccination is followed by the curve of deaths."

To understand the significance of his statement you need to understand the significance of his expertise. Professor Dr. Luc Montagnier has been called the world's leading virologist. He led the team that identified the human immunodeficiency virus (HIV) and shared half the 2008 Nobel Prize with his colleague Françoise Barré-Sinoussi. He has received numerous achievements and awards.

What he and Vanden Bossche are describing is called Antibody Dependent Enhancement. Dr. Montagnier echoes what has been said by Vanden Bossche. "We should never be vaccinated during an epidemic, and epidemiologists know this."

Those bullying us for refusing the jab are being manipulated because the truth is that the vaccinated have higher levels of the virus and are more likely to be infecting others. In one study, healthcare workers who have had the injection, for example, are 251 times more contagious than those who had not. Those who have received the shot are dangerous to those of us who have not taken it. They are also the ones responsible for the delta variant since their immune system is not killing the virus but giving it a safe place to evolve into a stronger strain.

Side effects of the transmission experienced by those who are near the vaccinated are more difficult to track. There's no formal database for those *not* vaccinated to log the abnormalities they are experiencing. We have no way of measuring the significance of the shots on those who have been transmitted upon by the vaccinated, but here are a few common effects that have been noted:

- Bleeding for weeks (women)
- Missed periods
- Post-menopausal bleeding
- Women passing large clots
- Pregnant women developing clots
- Miscarriages
- Breast irregularities
- Bloody noses
- Other clotting issues
- Bruising on the legs
- Swelling of genitals
- Decidual casts of women's uteruses being passed
- Erectile dysfunction

### The Hope is In the Resistance

There is hope for mankind from the continuously mutating virus that will now grow stronger because those vaccinated do not have an innate immune system to fight it. They no longer have NK cells that kill it nor nonspecific antibodies that finish the job. But, if enough of us refuse the vaccine *our* innate immune systems can fight the virus and create true herd immunity that saves mankind. The cure is in the resistance. Those of us refusing the jabs make up an army if we continue to resist.

The predictions Kimberly made in January 2016 came to pass. After reviewing the side effects of the vaccines and long-term outcomes that are possible, it appears that due to the increasing antigen loads that vaccine recipients will be creating a permanent change of the immune system change. She is now predicting that within 6 to 18 months, we will see a large percentage of the vaccinated begin to die. Most of them will die from lung damage as a result of massive inflammation. However, this appears as a lung infection which can also be confused with COVID or COVID pneumonia. This reaction can also be confused with a breakthrough infection. To keep the fear going and keep people coming back for more shots, the new infections that are the results of having had the first round of jabs will be reported as Covid. The media will blame those of us who are jab-free and people will turn on us.

*"People will oppress each other— man against man, neighbor against neighbor. Young people will insult their elders, and vulgar people will sneer at the honorable." Isaiah 3:5 (NLT)*

In the future we will see a massive death count that is misdiagnosed as a variant of the Covid virus followed by further lockdowns, restrictions of freedoms, travel restrictions and inevitably more vaccinations which will cause it all to repeat. Could it be that the push for vaccination has only just begun? Compliance doesn't work! This is why we had hats made for our patients that said, "Be the Resistance".

The Bible says in James 4:7, "So humble yourselves before God. Resist the devil and he will flee." (New King James Version) How do you resist? You resist by creating a body with an immune system to resist what comes your way. You resist by not putting your head in the sand and by getting the truth. You resist by not being silenced by Big Tech.

Maybe you're a person who is reading this and you already got the vaccine. You can still resist by taking care of your temple (your body) and not getting another one. You resist by telling the truth to your loved ones even if they don't want to hear it. Rosa Parks decided she wasn't going to sit in the back of the bus anymore. Some of you will have to decide if you will defy the Chemical Religion and set a precedent or will you go with the flow and hope it all works out in the end.

In the 1930's German citizens heard rumors of what was happening to people who did not fit the agenda, but they could not believe a government could do such a thing. Their denial and refusal to rise-up allowed the Nazi power to grow and brought death across the world.

A pandemic is what this has been called because its affects have stretched across the entire world. The World Health Organization and multiple governments are under the Chemical Religion's spell. In a sense we are dealing with a kind of world war again. This is not going to go away unless we resist. The sooner we come together, the fewer casualties we will suffer.

## Hospital Treated "COVID" Case January 2021

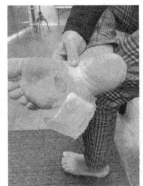
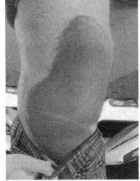
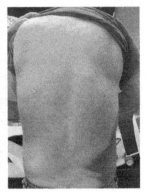

January 26          January 26          January 26

## After 1 Week under Dr. Erb's Care

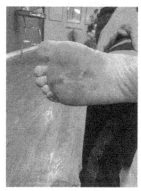

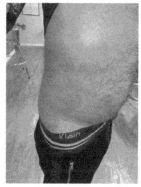

- 5 Adjustments
- 4 Hyperbaric Sessions
- Most Advanced Diet Plan
- Adding in Healing Supplements

Feb 2                    Feb 2

On January 6, 2021 our eldest son called me at midnight. He said his brother took their dad to the ER, but they weren't too worried about him. Knowing my ex-husband never went to the doctor, I was already concerned.

Piecing together what happened, I learned that Travis had taken two COVID tests, one was positive several days earlier, but the one he took that morning was negative. He didn't have anyone caring for him, so COVID developed into a bad case of pneumonia that he couldn't kick.

The next morning in the ER, Travis was feeling well enough to make several phone calls and order groceries to be delivered to his home. He never responded to my text and he stopped responding to the boys, who said the last they heard from him he was being transported to a hospital. Neither the ER nor the hospital contacted anyone, leaving us scrambling to find him. Our middle son remembered that he and his dad tracked each other's location on their phones, so we were able to see that he had been taken to a hospital nearly an hour away from us.

Feeling desperate, I called the hospital and pretended to be my ex-husband's wife. They said that they were just trying to find someone to call for permission to put in a PICC line. I wondered later why they were trying to open his phone to find someone to call when he had given an emergency contact number for someone they never bothered to call.

On the long drive to the hospital Travis remembered telling the medical drivers that he was cold. They refused to change the temperature or give him a blanket each time he pleaded. They just kept telling him they were almost there.

The boys' father left the ER well enough that they only planned to send him to be monitored in a lower-level unit. But when he arrived, he was shivering. This was a result from being left uncared for on the drive to the hospital. He began to panic, and his vitals were indicating the distress brought on by the admittance process. Without anyone's permission, the doctor put the man I had spent most my life with in the ICU. They sedated him, put him on paralysis, put a catheter in him and shoved a ventilator down his throat. If only I had called a little sooner, maybe I could have saved him from all that—and from what came next.

I asked the nurse what the dangers of a PICC line are since it was so important to get permission for that, especially considering they had already taken the liberty of putting Travis on a ventilator without permission. She said there was a small chance it could cause an infection. At this point I didn't feel I had much choice, so I agreed.

That night the boys and I drove to see their dad and assess the situation. He had been labeled COVID, so they were refusing to let us see him even though we had already had COVID and were still immune. We weren't going to catch it and we weren't going to pass it. I even explained that Travis had tested negative the morning before, so I was going to need to see documentation of their positive test. They handed me what they said was a positive test from the ER and a positive test they had performed. We later received confirmation from the ER that he had tested **negative**. Things were turning suspicious.

I told the staff I didn't know if I could feel comfortable continuing care unless we could see that he was okay, so the nurse convinced the doctor to come speak with me. The doctor explained his version of what happened, leaving many details out that I would discover later.

Knowing Travis had arrived coherent, I asked the doctor if his patient had given him permission to be put on a ventilator. Indignantly, he responded, "He would've died!" Knowing what I know now, it was very unlikely that a healthy mid-forties man who just needed antibiotics and care for his lungs was going to die if such extreme measures weren't inflicted upon him. He most likely needed rest, he needed a loved one for emotional support to be with him and he would've been out of there in a couple of days.

The doctor laughed at me when I suggested we get the ventilator off in three days. He insisted it would be at least two weeks. I had read about what happened in a New York hospital that kept putting COVID patients on ventilators for the money and losing them, but I held my tongue. The doctor brought up New York and assured me that he had only seen a 25% mortality rate on ventilators since COVID. That didn't make me feel any better about what my children's father was facing.

I spoke sternly and told the doctor that I was extremely uncomfortable with the ventilator and that I was going to need him to "aggressively pursue" getting it removed. And with that, the doctor agreed to let me see the man I had spent 20 years of my life with. He was covered in tubes and machines. It was the most helpless feeling seeing him like that and knowing we would not be able to stay with him. He would be left alone in a sterile environment.

I received updates every day. The numbers were moving quickly in the right direction, but they had one concern: Travis had begun to run a fever, indicating an infection. Once again, they needed my permission to put in another PICC line. That "small" chance of infection was now one more thing he was going to need to overcome.

The doctors seemed to be honoring my wish to get Travis off the ventilator, but the process didn't make sense. It was expected that the patient would first be removed from sedation before they take the scary and uncomfortable thing out. Travis remembered waking up many times feeling like he was fighting to keep the staff from putting this thing down his throat, not realizing that it was already in. Each time he would have to be immediately sedated again.

I explained to the doctor that this process wasn't going to work. After several conversations, they finally removed the ventilator before allowing the sedation to wear off. He was on the ventilator until January 19, 2021, just shy of two weeks, though his numbers indicated he could've been free sooner.

Waking from the medically induced coma, he had forgotten some of his life. He had to relive painful details as the sedation meds continued to wear off. While still so vulnerable, the doctors scared him, saying he would've died without them and threw out bloated numbers about COVID to make their patient feel grateful for how much was taken from him when they made the choice to put him on the ventilator. He had lost over 40 pounds and looked weak. He lost his strength and his health. He lost almost a month of his life.

His condition was downgraded, and he was moved to a different floor where a nurse would mistreat him. He also noticed that his foot was all wrapped up. No one would tell him what happened. The staff never mentioned it to me in our updates. He had a huge blister covering most of the bottom of his foot, making it nearly impossible to walk. They said that he's "a big man" and had pushed against a wall while he was in the induced coma. He's 5'9" and he was on paralysis (paralyzing meds), so their explanation doesn't make sense. It also sounded rehearsed as we asked other hospital staff.

Just when the boys and I were beginning to hold conversations with him, where their dad sounded mentally clearer, things got scary. He started hallucinating. The boys and I were worried. No one from the hospital was calling me with updates anymore and I couldn't get his nurse to return my calls. The nurse who answered the phone assured me that hallucinations are normal for COVID patients.

In desperation, I called down to the ICU and was able to speak with a nurse who knew us. He was kind enough to go upstairs and check on his former patient. He let me know that my Travis was being given a sleep medicine. Exhausted, I went to bed feeling better and decided I'd research the med in the morning. It turns out the drug was an antidepressant and was "not to be used as a first resort sleep aid." Also, the instructions for use warned to call your doctor immediately if a patient began hallucinating. In our case, we couldn't get the doctor to call back.

I was able to catch Travis at a clear moment and warned him to stop taking the pill. He was bullied a bit by the nurse, but he was growing stronger and stood his ground.

The hospital was preparing for his release, but first he had to agree to go to physical therapy. They were recommending inpatient care and found a place closer to us that allowed two visitors a day over the age of 18 years. Our youngest son would not get to see his dad for another three weeks. The lady I spoke to said that most patients stay two weeks, but because his insurance is so good, he'd stay for three. When I asked what happens if a patient decides he wants to go home sooner, she warned that it would be against doctor's orders, and he could have an issue with his insurance. We were beginning to feel like prisoners, not patients, being detained without rights.

The kids' father decided he'd recover most quickly going to Erb Family Wellness, where he would receive daily spinal adjustments, hyperbaric treatments, infrared sauna sessions and supplements to restore and rebuild his body. He'd be able to eat healthy, high-quality food of his choice and sleep in his own bed at night.

As you can imagine, the hospital didn't approve, and they began to bully Travis more. They insisted on driving him to his first appointment, where we could meet him and approve of the facility. I wondered how much that drive would've cost insurance?

When he continued to resist their recommendations, a nurse snidely asked, "Do you have $40,000 dollars laying around for in home care?" She was silenced when he answered, "yes." Insurance and the medical profession would like us to believe it's too expensive to get care outside of their system when, in reality, their system cost the father of my children something more valuable than money, and it nearly cost him his life.

We brought Travis home January 26th. He began to get his life back. He spent time with his kids, drove himself around and went back to the office. His foot is still aching, which isn't a symptom from COVID but of hospital negligence. It's been a lingering reminder of the care he received from the hospital and a source of painful humbling. He walked with a limp as we toured our son's future college, led by the strong football coaches. Fatigued and suffering with each step, he tried to keep up, though he recognized that the group had dropped back for his sake.

After watching the once strong, proud man hurt all day, I came home determined to find out what really happened to his foot. I discovered that it was medical neglect. Not only had it caused the pressure ulcers on his foot, but the negligence had also put him at risk for other more dangerous issues.

I found a study from 1995 that said patients who are unable to move themselves need to be adjusted 9.9 times per shift to avoid the effects of "migration." Positioning the head of the bed above a 30-degree angle reduces the risk of VAP (ventilator-associated pneumonia). Wait, what?! He was there to be treated for pneumonia and he was put on a device that could actually cause pneumonia!

The article written for nurses caring for patients on ventilators and otherwise incapacitated warned that to avoid kyphosis, a condition that reduces lung capacity, Travis needed to remain properly elevated. Again, he was being treated for his sick lungs with the goal of increasing his lung capacity for recovery, but clearly his needs were being neglected as evidenced by the pressure ulcers on his foot.

I discovered in another article written for medical staff caring for immobilized patients that there are four stages of pressure ulcers that can be caused when patients slide down and their feet are pressed against the end of the bed. The first stage can be detected by redness even if the patient is unable to express the pain and itching feeling being experienced. Travis walked out of the hospital with all the symptoms and evidence of stage four pressure ulcers, which is most often treated with surgery.

There are still so many questions left to be answered. Why was my sons' father taken to a hospital so far away? We never got a straight answer, but a stammering doctor suggesting maybe his hospital was the closest one with a bed. Why didn't they call the emergency contact person on their paperwork when they moved him? Or before they put a ventilator on him? Or when they wanted to put a PICC line in? Why did his nurse refuse to respond to my concerned calls? Why did they lie that the ER had tested him positive for COVID? Why did they refuse to retest him for COVID so we could see him while he was recovering at the hospital? Why were the medical staff so against us receiving after care outside of their system? They threatened not to release him if they didn't approve of our choice.

We may never have answers, but we are thankful that we got Travis out of that prison alive. Travis stood strong against the hospital bullying and we took him to Erb Family wellness. He was adjusted and spent time in the hyperbaric chamber.

We're thankful for the Erbs, who were able to begin to restore his health and his mental clarity. And we are thankful that the care he received from them was nothing near the $40, 000 that the nurse implied it would be. – Rebecca

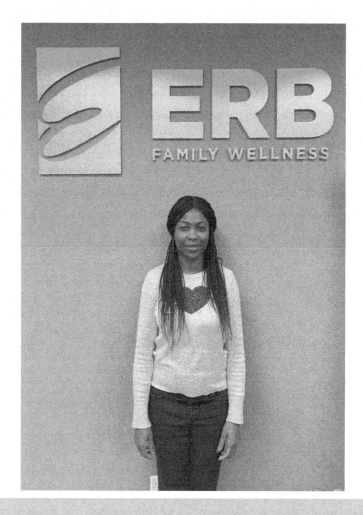

I have not eaten on the left side of my mouth in 12 years! After my first adjustment with Dr. David, my TMJ was corrected. I didn't realize my mouth had been misaligned and that it could be corrected with chiropractic treatment.

About a month or two ago I was recovering from COVID, but I had the worst cough. It wouldn't go away! I went to Erb Family Wellness for help and they recommended the hyperbaric treatment. That knocked the cough out in two sessions. – Temi Talabi

# CHAPTER 13
# CHOOSE LIFE!

"Today I have given you the choice between life and death,
between blessings and curses. Now I call on heaven and earth to
witness the choice you make. Oh, that you would choose life,
so that you and your descendants might live!"

Deuteronomy 30:19 NLT

God created our bodies to heal. When we get a cut, our skin regrows. When we consume something toxic our innate filtration system protects us from poisoning. When we break a bone, it grows back together. Our bodies are intricately designed to recover on their own.

God never needed our help when it comes to healing our body. We just need to stop interfering with His design. We interfere when we manipulate our body's natural process with pharmaceuticals. We interfere with poor eating habits. And subluxation interferes with our perfectly created central nervous system that encompasses the entire function of our body.

God did His job when He created us. Our natural healing process is an absolute miracle! *Our* job is to remove anything that interferes with the power that enables our body to heal itself.

Keeping in mind that preventable medical error is the third leading cause of death in the U.S. (225,000 deaths a year), it seems clear that the greater health risk comes in putting our faith in the Chemical Religion.

Believe me when I say that we do not mean to attack doctors, nurses or healthcare workers. There are so many with us in the fight against the Chemical Religion's agenda. They want to protect their patients and see them recover. We are just saying that medicine and surgery should be used for emergency medical crisis when we need them. Do you really think we need more drugs to be healthy? Are our headaches because we are not taking enough ibuprofen? Preventative measures are being ignored and measures that come with life-altering and deadly consequences are being relied upon instead. God *formed* and man *deformed;* we're trying to *transform* and *reform,* bringing us back to God's original plan.

The Chemical Religion is a fast-paced movement with ever-growing numbers. More deaths, more lawsuits and more studies expose the increased health risks with pharmaceutical drug use. The numbers grow as more drugs are introduced and as updated studies are performed. We have done our best to keep up with those ever-evolving numbers as we wrote this book. We've been careful to back up those numbers with references. But Big Pharma and Big Tech are removing many of those references faster than we can type. Don't be surprised if you look one up and it's been deleted or revised to conform to the Chemical Religion's lies.

The following numbers were updated as of January 31st, 2020:

### Top Ten Biggest Pharma Lawsuits by Settlement Amount:

10. Amgen – $762m

9. Bayer and Johnson & Johnson – $775m

8. TAP Pharmaceutical – $875m

7. Merck – $950m

6. Eli Lilly and Company – $1.4bn

5. Abbott Laboratories – $1.5bn

4. Johnson & Johnson – $2.2bn

3. Pfizer – $2.3bn

2. Takeda Pharmaceutical – $2.4bn

1. GlaxoSmithKline – $3bn

Notice that America's trusted COVID vaccine makers listed. It's like taking a shot in the dark. What could possibly go wrong? I'd rather take my chances with God's healing design: how about you? Are you ready to unplug from the Chemical Religion and plug into true healing? Get ready to be empowered by five simple practices that will change your health and change your life. Let's get started!

## The Gospels of Good Health

We have Good News that sets free those taken captive by the Chemical Religion. Health was God's plan from the beginning, and He made it pretty simple. The Gospels of Good Health are:

1.  Hope-filled Mind
2.  Tap Into God's Power Source
3.  Get Back to the Garden
4.  Breath in Energy
5.  Repent of Toxins

Thomas Edison predicted, "The doctor of the future will give no medicine but will interest his patient in the care of the human frame, in diet and in the cause and prevention of disease." We are the doctors of the future. Others are rising up as well to bring healthcare back to the basics.

We're going to explain how focusing on these five areas will keep you physically thriving. No diagnoses. No doctors telling you, "It's just old age." No surgeries. No meds.

## Hope-filled Mind

According to Google, "Hope is a feeling of expectation and desire for a certain thing to happen." It's what drives us to keep looking for answers when circumstances aren't going our way. Hope keeps us afloat through life's storms if we hang on to it relentlessly, but sometimes our hands begin to burn as it's being ripped from our grip. Letting go starts to feel like it'll hurt less than being disappointed again.

The Bible says, "Hope deferred makes the heart sick." By the time many of our patients get to us they've tried a lot of treatments that have failed them. They walk in and we can tell pretty quickly who is going to overcome their health hurdle and who will need to take hold of the hope they've lost first.

Hopelessness is cancer in the mind that spreads throughout the body. People's ability to keep expecting good regardless of what they're facing is foundational for overall health. The Bible says that the power of life and death are in our words and our words flow from our thoughts. That's why, at our offices, we treat hopelessness first. From the moment our patients walk through our doors they are met with our tagline: "The greatest place of hope and healing!" We aren't scared by their diagnosis. We've seen everything from cancer to infertility have to flee when truth is shared and applied.

If you are feeling hopeless, repentance is the place to start. Repentance simply means *to turn away from*. Turn away from the darkness and turn to Jesus who is the light of the world. He is the Great Physician, and He loves you so much. Turn away from entertainment forms that depress and from friends who bring you down. Find a Spirit-filled church with people who will encourage you. Switch off the bad news and switch on the good news of Christ! Then let Him begin a good work in you that He promises to complete. These are a few places to start, but we will share some more encouragements below.

## Landing After Fight-or-Flight

Every morning, before we open our doors, we start our day in prayer. Our patients are our family, our tribe. We know the health issues they are each fighting, and we know the kinds of things they are facing in life. Some have children who have gone astray. Others are wondering if they will soon lose their jobs. We recognize that the stress they face each day affects their overall health.

Have you heard the statement, "fight-or-flight?" When faced with danger or stress, it is your body's natural physiological reaction to what's called "the acute stress response."

I'm sure you've had an experience, for example, when you hear a loud sound or encounter a frightening situation. Maybe your kids play a joke on you and jump out at you, what happens to your body?

Your hormones kick in, prompting the release of adrenaline and cortisol. Adrenaline increases your heart rate, elevates your blood pressure and boosts energy supplies (so you can run if you need to). Cortisol, the primary stress hormone, increases glucose in the bloodstream, enhances your brain's use of glucose and increases the availability of substances that repair tissues.

Cortisol also curbs functions that would be nonessential or detrimental in a fight-or-flight situation. It alters immune system responses and suppresses the digestive system, the reproductive system and growth processes. This natural alarm system communicates with regions of your brain that control mood, motivation and fear.

The body's stress-response system is usually self-limiting; after the perceived threat has passed, everything returns to normal. Your adrenaline and cortisol levels drop, your heart rate and blood pressure return to baseline levels, and other systems resume their regular activities.

A problem arises when you're experiencing prolonged stress that keeps you in fight-or-flight mode. The effects from high levels of adrenaline and cortisol wreak havoc on your body. You may experience panic attacks from the rapid heart rate and lasting heightened blood pressure is certainly not a good thing, either.

Like many of our patients, you may have experienced prolonged stress from the pandemic and have gained weight. We call that the "Quarantine Fifteen." The constant glucose released from cortisol increases belly fat. Depression, fatigue, adrenal burnout, reduced immunity and slowed metabolism are more effects that come with living in a state of mental stress.

We're hearing of individuals who are doing all the right things to lose the weight but are struggling. Don Clum is a Chiropractor, a functional fitness expert and a specialist in Advanced Metabolic Nutrition. He emphasizes that, "There's no amount of protein you could take or diet restrictions you could implement that will make you lose weight if your hormones are out of sync." That's why it's so important to your health and your waistline to find a way to bring your stress levels down.

If not before, 2020 has definitely shown us it's impossible to avoid stress all together. But that doesn't mean all hope is lost. There are some practices that can help get us through. Chiropractic adjustments can be helpful in reducing stress. They release muscle tension, soothe irritated spinal nerves and improve blood circulation. Easing these subluxation symptoms can often alert the brain to switch off the fight-or-flight response so your body can return to a more relaxed state. It's like a massage for your central nervous system. Achieving a balanced spine is a crucial element of managing personal stress.

One thing is true. "It came to pass ..." The Bible speaks of many uncertain times stating that they came to pass. No storm ever lasts forever, but what happens when the Shepherd leads us beside still waters when there's still a tempest in our head?

Did you know that the fight-or-flight response can be triggered by both real and imaginary threats? That's why what we think about is often as important as what we experience. What we think about determines our beliefs. Our thoughts become our reality. The scenarios we play out can either take us down a dark road that fuels fear and anxiety or one of hope in a faithful God who will get us through. "You will keep him in perfect peace, whose mind is stayed on You, because he trusts in You." Isaiah 26:3 NKJV

Meditating on scripture is a great way to overcome toxic thought patterns that lead to hopelessness, stress, anxiety and depression. The Bible puts it like this: "And do not be conformed to this world, but be transformed by the *renewing of your mind*, that you may prove what is that good and acceptable and perfect will of God." Romans 12:2 NKJV

Most of our internal stressors come from our own thoughts and beliefs. We have the ability to manage these, but sometimes we become plagued by worry, anxiety, uncertainty, fears and other forms of negativity. It feels like everywhere we turn we are faced with opposition. In those seasons we may begin to form new thought processes that are focused on negative expectations and emotions. Or maybe we have never been in the habit of believing the best and thinking about whatsoever is of good report (as the Bible puts it). Our old way of thinking, before we knew God or after the battle that beat us down must be transformed.

We renew our minds with the truth and truth is found in scripture. Meditate on what is good and positive. "Casting down imaginations, and every high thing that is exalted against the knowledge of God and *bringing every thought into captivity to the obedience of Christ*," 2 Corinthians 7:5 American Standard Version.

If you are struggling with depression, find someone who can help you navigate your way through the cloud. A good therapist will point you to Christ, not to meds.

## Stress By Subluxation

Believe it or not, chiropractors can help you find your way out of the darkness, too. The part of your brain that deals with your emotions is the part of your brain most affected by subluxation. Why are so many of our patients able to get off their emotional meds after getting regular corrective adjustments?

Besides the fact that subluxation affects your serotonin levels which can cause depression, long-term stress alters internal chemistry with the flood of the hormones cortisol and adrenaline just like in fight-or-flight.

One of the effects of chronic stress is muscle tension and contraction, which can lead to uneven pressure on the skeleton, which in turn leads to subluxation. It is a dangerous cycle. Stress causes subluxation and subluxation causes stress. That's another reason, besides the immune boost they give, that getting routine adjustments even after you are symptom free is important.

The Gospels of Good Health are all connected like a puzzle that needs each piece to complete the picture. Besides holding onto hope and spinal adjustments to manage or overcome stress, we'll show you how what you eat, getting exercise and avoiding toxins all play a part too. Just like we're made up of body, mind and spirit and each operates separately yet all operate and function together, so it is with the Gospels of Good Health.

## Turn Your Power On The Central Nervous System

Before David's heart scare, we were once chiropractors who were not taught about subluxation. Unfortunately, many other chiropractors are giving nonspecific adjustments the way we had done. If we had not met the D.C who taught us about treating subluxation, we too would still be giving adjustments that do not correct interference of the central nervous system. That's why it's important to ask two questions when looking for a chiropractor.

1. Do you treat subluxations?

2. Do you take before and after treatment x-rays?

Whether you're facing cancer, heart disease or any other health condition (in the words of Hippocrates), "Look well to the spine for the cause of disease." Don't look for a diagnosis, look for the cause to bring correction.

This is one of the most important things that you will ever learn regarding how to be happy, healthy and to remain thriving for your kids and your grandkids. As doctors we get asked all the time, "What's the most important thing I can do for my health?" People wonder if it's exercise. Is it nutrition? Is it all about the supplements they take?

To measure the importance each element bears upon your body, you simply need to think about how long your body can survive without each. How long can you go without food? If you've ever seen Survivor, you know that you can go a couple of *weeks* without food. How long can you go without water? You can only go a couple of *days* without water. That means water is more essential than food. But air is actually even more important than food and water. How long can you go without air? You can only survive a couple *minutes* without oxygen. Air is actually more important than food or water, but there's one thing that's even more important than these three. People don't usually think about the importance of their nerve supply. Nerve supply is the missing link when it comes to wellness.

How long can you go without proper nerve supply? If I cut your spinal cord in half, what happens to you? You're dead. Immediately. You cannot go one *second* without proper nerve supply. More important than exercise (that increases oxygen consumption) and more important than nutrition is maintaining a healthy, balanced central nervous system.

You remember Christopher Reeves, right? Christopher Reeves fell off the horse, and what did he damage? He damaged his spinal cord. It shut down everything in his body. If I gave Christopher Reeves a really good nutrition plan, he wasn't going to get better. If I gave him a really good detox plan, he wasn't going to get better. He wasn't going to get better because he had broken his spine and it severed his spinal cord. The spinal cord could no longer carry blood, oxygen or signals from the brain to the rest of his body. He lost mobility, but his organs also began to die like plants without water and sunlight.

In our offices, after adjusting patients' spines, we like to announce, "Your power is on!" That's because your nervous system controls all health and healing in your body. Where does that nerve supply come from? It comes from your brain and your spinal cord; they control everything that happens in your entire body. For your heart to beat, for your lungs to breathe, for your food to digest, for your cortisol levels to work properly; information must go from your brain down your spinal cord through these nerves. If it's properly functioning at 100% then all of those other things like nutrition and exercise will further promote your body's immune response. If it's not functioning optimally, it's like a light switch that doesn't work because the fuse box needs to be reset. This is called subluxation.

## The Effects of Subluxation

How do you know if your spine is subluxated? There are warning signs, and thank God there are, because how much would it be worth to know that your heart is malfunctioning before you have a heart attack? How much would it be worth to know that you're having things like constipation or IBS or things that have been shown to be precursors to colon cancer? How much is it worth to know that you're developing these things before you're actually in the hospital being told they have to take three feet out of your colon?

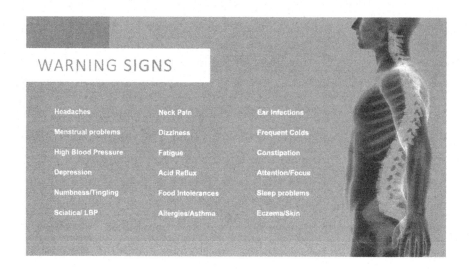

Subluxation will lead to degeneration in virtually every part of the body, depending on where in the spine it's occurring. The nervous system controls **everything.**

Look at the image of the spine below. It's like a map. You can follow with your finger from between each vertebra to the organs that are fed from the nerve running to them. Damaging the nerves in your spine can happen from car accidents, birth trauma or even from sitting on a computer all day long. When your spine gets shifted out of position it's called subluxation. Sitting on computers all day or teens looking down at their phones for hours a day cause "forward head posture" which is where the head begins to shift forward disrupting the natural curve in the spine and causing headaches. I'd say of 100 people who walk in with headaches probably 99 of them walk out with relief when we find the cause of their problem after a full exam. This shift literally crushes the nerves in your neck and will take decades off your life. This has been proven in the following studies and more.

- "Decreased blood flow from abnormal posture is a major factor in **all disease**, including cancer." *Reich, MD*

- Faulty posture (loss of curve in neck) causes weak immune system, organ disease, muscle tension and increased sensitivity to pain.

- A loss or increase in spinal curves increases mortality (speeds up death) and **takes up to 14 years off your life**.

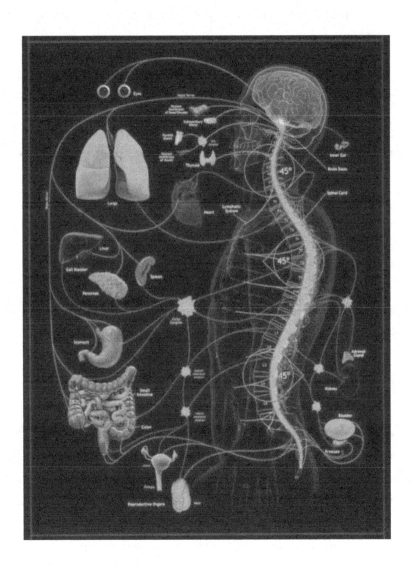

The Journal of Manipulative and Physiologic Therapeutics did a study that evaluated 311 chiropractic patients, aged 65 and older. Each had received "maintenance care" for five years or longer versus healthy citizens the same age. Their discoveries have served to further fuel our passion for chiropractic care.

- Chiropractic patients spent only 31% of the national average for health care
- They had 50% fewer medical provider visits
- Their health habits were radically better then overall populations
- They had far less cigarette consumption
- 98.5% believed that care to be considerably or extremely valuable
- They had 60.2% fewer hospital admissions
- They had 59% less days hospitalized
- They had 62% less outpatient surgeries
- They had 85% less pharmaceutical costs

In the *Journal of Hypertension*, they found that chiropractic adjustments lowered blood pressure better than the drugs HCTZ and Lisinopril.

**Spinal Alignment is Needed for Digestion and Absorption of Nutrients**

What use is the best food in the world if your body can't digest, absorb or assimilate it? Subluxation is why one child can eat McDonalds and sugar and rarely be sick, yet another eats gluten free, organic and raw yet is ridden with allergies, asthma and eczema. It doesn't matter how clean you eat if you have interference in your central nervous system. A balanced spine is a crucial element to your brain properly communicating with your gut and stimulation of your digestion.

The gut and brain use their shared neurotransmitters, including acetylcholine and serotonin, to transmit information back and forth by way of the sympathetic and parasympathetic nerves.

Interference in the gut-brain communication caused by spinal misalignment hinders digestion, and in turn, one's ability to properly absorb nutrients. Plus, the signals received from the brain trigger one to eat and stop eating, helping to avoid overconsumption.

Subluxation affects your serotonin levels, which can cause depression, insomnia, fatigue and acid reflux. Nexium, the purple pill that's prescribed for acid reflux, interferes with the body's ability to heal. It isn't fixing the problem; it's adding to it.

The same is true with any of the medications you might take. If you have an issue caused by subluxation and you take a medication for it, it's like putting a piece of duct tape over the check engine light. It doesn't fix anything! If you keep driving your car like that, it's going to blow up. Can you see that if you keep ignoring these warning signs, here comes heart disease, cancer or diabetes? Cover up these symptoms and you're going to blow a gasket.

## Get Back to the Garden

Since man was kicked out of the Garden of Eden for choosing food that God said would bring death, humans have continued to crave what feeds their lusts for pleasure over their need for nutrition. **Food by God** fills and heals. **Food by Man** bloats and blocks. It causes inflammation, it blocks arteries and keeps our body in a state of constantly trying to recover.

God pointed out some meats that we should avoid and others that he referred to as "clean." Leviticus and Deuteronomy require that all animals and animal byproducts that do not chew the cud and do not have cloven hoofs (such as pigs and horses) should not be eaten, along with fish without fins and scales, shellfish such as clams, oysters, shrimp, crabs or any other creature creeping across the ocean's floor. Vultures, hawks, owls and herons are also on God's avoid list, along with the blood of any animal. All foods outside these categories were permissible for consumption. *Clean eating* has become a catchphrase in the fitness industry- and God literally invented the term. It just goes to show that His Word is forever relevant.

We realize that in our new covenant with Christ these meats are no longer forbidden, but that doesn't mean they are suddenly healthy. There was a reason God forbade them. In First Corinthians 6:12 AMP it's better explained as, "Everything is permissible for me, but not all things are beneficial. Everything is permissible for me, but I will not be enslaved by anything [and brought under its power, allowing it to control me]." If we allow our fleshly desires to drive our appetites, we will reap the consequences.

In Chapter Two we shared about the Forbidden Fruit of our day. The serpent in *our* garden is tempting us with genetically modified foods containing poisons like glyphosate. It's tempting us with the convenience of processed foods. That's where we went into more details about what to eat and what to avoid, but here are a few refreshers. In the Appendix we provide you with an easily accessible reference of toxins.

**Simply Stated:**

- Fresh is best.
- Packaged is poor.
- Artificial and unnatural are inedible.
- Fat is fine.
- Can't read it, don't eat it.

**What to Look For:**

- BPA-free – Does not contain the industrial chemical BPA

- Non-GMO – Verifies it does not contain genetically modified organisms.

- USDA Organic – Organic products meeting the USDA requirements.

**What to Eat:**

- Stevia or erythritol instead of sugar or artificial sweeteners

- Low glycemic fruits like berries, grapefruit and granny smith apples

- Grass-fed, free-range, not corn fed, antibiotic/GH free beef, bison, chicken, eggs

- Non-farm raised fish

- Quality whey protein from 100% naturally raised cows

- No hormones or pesticides

- Good fats such as olive oil, coconut oil, avocados, nuts (such as walnuts and almonds) and omega 3 fatty acids

Read labels and don't be fooled by deceptive marketing. You are what you eat.

## When Food isn't Enough

Our soil has been abused and depleted of nutrients so that the produce we grow today contains far less nutrients than it did in our grandparents' gardens. Thankfully God planned ahead and created ways to increase our vitamin intake through specific foods and herbs.

There are a lot of supplements out there. It can be overwhelming walking through the aisles of immune boosters, sleep remedies, vitamins and minerals. One week everyone is talking about turmeric and another week ginger is all the rage. We rush to purchase another super-food to stay up with the trends. Our cabinets can become filled with really great vitamins and herbs, but it might become overwhelming taking them all.

What if there was a way to give your body only what it's missing? What if you didn't have to guess? Metabolic testing will show you what your body needs so you won't be too full to eat *actual* food after you've swallowed all those healthy pills.

Metabolic testing is an advanced test that uses blood, urine and saliva to determine many risk factors such as cancer, autoimmune disease and digestive disorders. It can tell you what your body is missing and can even give indicators to what kinds of toxins you are being exposed. The Appendix has our contact information if you need help finding a place that offers the testing.

Our family tests regularly to ensure we stay on top of our environment. If we see any markers in our results indicating that we are headed for a storm, we don't fill prescriptions. We don't run to the grocery store's vitamin section, either. We research products containing the most potent and absorbable ingredients without additives. You get what you pay for. Health doesn't come from bargain shopping.

## Breathe In Energy

Another important piece of the puzzle is a breath of fresh air. Oxygen is life to our cells, and it makes sense. When God formed man out of dust, Adam didn't come to life until the Maker first blew into his lungs.

This is one "supplement" that is pretty cheap, and we can get it in bulk by exercising. Physical activity increases our heart rate and forces our lungs to suck in more air. So, take the stairs and stop looking for that parking spot by the front entrance.

In Chapters Five and Seven we talked about some of the benefits of exercise, but its value needs to be restated. Exercise helps to reduce symptoms of stress, anxiety, depression and obsessive-compulsive disorder.

"Deep breathing techniques which increase oxygen to the cell are the most important factors in living a disease free and energetic life ..." encouraged Otto Warburg, President, Institute of Cell Physiology, Nobel Prize Winner.

**Exercise Improves:**

- Digestion

- Mood

- Metabolism

- Cognitive function

- Sleep quality

**It Decreases Risk of:**

- Chronic diseases

- Senility

- Dementia

Exercise also promotes the growth of new nerve cells, which protect from Alzheimer's and other memory related diseases. Exercise induces the release of beneficial proteins in the brain. These nourishing proteins keep brain cells (also known as neurons) healthy and promote the growth of new neurons. So, let's get our bodies moving and sucking in that air!

### Hyperbaric Treatment

The only thing better than breathing in more air is breathing in more *quality* air. Our environment is filled with pollutants, but we discovered a way to fill our lungs with oxygen that has some of the same benefits contained in the air before the fall of man.

Hyperbaric therapy is a medical treatment that enhances the body's natural healing process. While lying comfortably on an enclosed bed, patients inhale oxygen where atmospheric pressure is increased and controlled. It is used for a wide variety of treatments usually as a part of an overall medical care plan. Mild Hyperbaric Oxygen Therapy saturates body fluids, tissues and cells with oxygen under pressure. Many of the benefits are listed here:

- Stroke and Heart Attack Prevention & Treatment
- Increase Natural Killer Cell Activity and Function
- Sports injuries
- Cancer Prevention and Treatment
- Diabetes
- Reduces Gastrointestinal Issues
- Decreases Inflammation & Pain
- Enhances Nutritional Absorption
- Increases Collagen Production
- Promotes Optimal Blood Flow
- Reduces Paralysis
- Stimulates the Creation of Blood Vessels to Reclaim Damaged Brain Tissue
- Helps Improve Ulcerative Colitis
- Improves Sleep Pattern
- Reduces Risk of Infection
- Stimulated the Creation of New Stem Cells
- Improves Blood Flow
- Increases Energy Levels
- Promotes the Creation of New Brain Cells
- Escalates the Creation of New Brain Connections
- Alleviates Spasticity
- Lessens Frequency of Seizures
- Minimizes Oxidative Stress
- Enhance Memory and Mental Performance
- Develops & Regains Cognitive/Motor Functions
- Accelerated growth & repair of damaged tissue
- Facilitates the Formation of New Brain Connections
- Improves Vision and Speech
- Neurodegenerative
- Conditions (Alzheimer's, Parkinson's, Huntington's Disease)
- Accelerates Tissue Repair and Healing
- Combats Cellulitis
- Reduces Tendinitis
- Remediates Inflammatory Bowel Disease
- Remediates Arthritis
- Increases Serotonin Levels

- Neurological Injuries
  (Stroke, Traumatic Brain
  & Spinal Cord Injuries,
  Concussions)
- Improves Concentration

- Neurodevelopment
  Conditions (Autism,
  Cerebral Palsy, Fetal
  Alcohol Syndrome)

Our website contains much more about the benefits and surprising diseases hyperbaric therapy has been shown to improve. Visit us at Erbfamilyhyperbaric.com.

Oxygen is so essential to the body that you can only go minutes without it. It's inexpensive, and your supply can be increased by including exercise in your lifestyle. So, breathe in energy!

## Repent from Toxins

We all do our best to care for and protect our families as we wipe away the germs and feed them meals from boxes with clever advertisements. But we may be wiping on more toxic substances and spoon feeding our babies sickness. The Appendix offers a list of household hazards to avoid. Chapter Two explains the dangers contained in common foods found in the American pantry. In this chapter we want to challenge you to replace those toxins found in your cleaning products, cosmetics, personal hygiene products and detergents. Look for ingredients like essential oils that have cleaning properties in them. Search out websites that keep up with ingredients as trusted brands often fall into the wrong hands.

Toxins are everywhere! Thankfully, God designed our bodies to overcome and to heal when we come in contact with them. He did His job, but we must remember to be diligent to do ours. Do you remember what our part is in taking care of our body? Our job is to remove the interference. Turning away from toxins is a huge step! But not all toxins come from things that we consume or that can be avoided.

Electromagnetic field (EMF) radiation is an immunosuppressant, which means it disables your immune system's ability to respond to foreign substances. Subjection comes through electronic devices such as cell phones, microwaves and laptops. Depending on the level of exposure, your body cannot combat toxins, bacteria, viruses and chemicals like mold and pesticides that infiltrate it to the same degree, if at all. You can find more information about EMFs in Chapter Six and in the Appendix, but in this chapter, we want to tell you how you can protect yourself from the harm they inflict.

Some M.D.s have begun to treat patients by helping them to eliminate their exposure to EMFs. Dr. Dietrich Klinghardt, M.D., PHD., has his patients remove cordless telephones and turn off fuses at night. He found that reducing EMFs was more successful in treating Lyme Disease than any antibiotics he had tried.

We grew up without computers and we talked on a phone that was attached to the kitchen wall. The only smart thing about our phones were their ability to connect to an answering box that allowed friends to leave a message. Our children are growing up in a world that would collapse without technology. We've all come to rely on it so heavily that it would be impossible to completely cleanse ourselves from our devices. But what if we could protect ourselves from them?

EMF radiation shielding blocks the harmful waves being emitted from reaching your body.

A study evaluated 64 people with a variety of chronic diseases. For eight hours a day they blocked EMF exposure resulting in 90% of the patients experiencing a "definite" or "strong" improvement in their symptoms.

Another step you can take to protect yourself from EMF exposure is to reduce the time you're connected to these devices. Don't feel like you're a strict parent because you're limiting your children's time as well. Set an example to them and put on *your* oxygen mask, so to speak, first. That's a rule across the board when it comes to living a healthy lifestyle. Children often duplicate the habits of their parents. If you are overweight, have digestive problems, allergies or diabetes chances are your children will develop these issues over time as well. Lead and they will likely follow.

Limiting your connection time isn't enough. When you aren't using a device, make sure to turn it off completely. Even when your phone is locked or your laptop has gone to sleep, devices still emit EMF radiation. Setting a device to Airplane Mode will turn off its radio signal and protect you. Also remember to turn off your Wi-Fi router before bed since you won't need it until morning. Taking it one step further, it's a good idea to keep electronic devices out of the bedroom. Go get yourself an old-fashioned alarm clock to replace your phone alarm.

Turn away from the things that interfere with God's design. Let the fever do its job rather than trying to control it. Let the cholesterol do its job rather than trying to eliminate it. Get waivers from your state so you won't have to vaccinate. Trust God's process.

## Cleanse Yourself

"Therefore, since we have these [great and wonderful] promises, beloved, let us cleanse ourselves from everything that contaminates body and spirit, completing holiness [living a consecrated life—a life set apart for God's purpose] in the fear of God."

2 Corinthians 7:1 AMP

When you have done your best to turn away from toxins, it's time to cleanse yourself from them. Every day we bathe, we brush our teeth and we put on clean clothes. We keep our largest organ, our skin, washed, but what about cleaning our inner organs? Our kidneys, our liver, gallbladder and colon need washed too. Our environment is full of yuck that we ingest even with our most diligent effort to rid ourselves of them. If they get *on* our skin, they get *under* our skin as well.

Your everyday cleansing practice, like your daily shower, should include hydration. Drink plenty of water to avoid dehydration, which protects your kidneys by flushing out the toxins from them. Your kidneys also help filter blood before sending it back your heart. Blood pumps life throughout all your vital organs. Keeping it pure may be even more important than brushing your teeth every day.

Juicing is another practice you can add to your daily routine. It has many benefits besides feeding your cells and cleansing your blood. Just be careful you aren't filling your machine with a bunch of high sugar fruits. Bananas, melons, pears, grapes are fine in moderation but blueberries, strawberries and blackberries (to name a few) are lower glycemic. Add some greens and lemon juice with your berries. You can throw in some ginger and turmeric for a super nutritional boost. Get creative and make it fun with new recipes.

Relaxing in an infrared sauna is another way to get clean on the inside. Sweat out those toxins while you take some time to read, meditate or to just get a little time to yourself. It offers relief from arthritis, chronic fatigue syndrome, fibromyalgia, sports injuries and other chronic pain conditions. According to the Journal of the American Medical Association, regular use of a sauna compares to the same cardiovascular effect of running.

- A January 2009 study in Clinical Rheumatology showed that infrared saunas gave significant relief for patients with chronic pain such as rheumatoid arthritis.

- A recent study published in Internal Medicine, showed that patients with chronic pain saw their pain levels drop by nearly 70% after their first session of infrared sauna therapy.

There is a long list of benefits:

- Fights cellulite
- Relaxation

- Clear and tighter skin
- Improved circulation

- Relief from joint pain such as arthritis
- Weight loss
- Relief from sore muscles
- Detoxification

- Help ~~for~~ people with chronic fatigue syndrome
- Cleanses the liver
- Cleanses the gallbladder
- May help reduce blood pressure

In your family begin a culture of cleansing. Besides adding the practice to your hygienic routine, begin a yearly practice of cleansing for parasites, gallbladder, colon, kidneys and liver. Do your research or call our offices to find the best cleanses. You can also visit ErbFamilyDetox.com for more information

## Get Tested

Remember how we explained the dangers of radiation exposure that comes from routine mammograms? Well, that doesn't mean that you shouldn't be checked routinely. There are a lot of great nonmainstream tests out there. There are smart ways to stay on top of your health, one of which is thermography testing.

MRIs, X-rays and other scans tell us about body structure and thermography tell us about function of glands, organs and the immune system. I use thermography with my patients to gain insight into where their body is out of balance and what glands and organs need support. We use it for early detection, to identify root causes of illness and to guide and monitor these:

- Breasts
- Ovaries
- Uterus
- Heart
- Thyroid
- Teeth

- Colon
- Kidney
- Prostate
- Liver
- Gallbladder
- Pancreas

- Lymph
- Sinus
- Spinal Column
- Stomach
- Small Intestine

The thermography machine measures 120 specific points located on the face and torso. Then the body is exposed to cool air for ten minutes. The same points are re-measured after the ten minutes to see how each organ regulated under the stress of the cool down. The organs' ability to regulate provides information about the cellular and metabolic function or dysfunction. With the AlfaSight thermography machine, we can see what the body is doing before it becomes dysfunctional. You can visit us at ErbFamilyThermography.com for more information.

**What Do You Choose?**

We've given you the truth, putting you in the driver's seat. No more duct taping over symptoms in your engine. No more leaving your health in the hands of the Chemical Religion. Rip off the scales and learn how to be your own advocate. Read, learn, study and question the things you've researched.

It's scary when the beliefs we have grown up with are challenged. But a paradigm shift can be liberating when it's founded in truth. Truth empowers and empowered people don't fear. You are now empowered with the Good News. The Gospels of Good Health will set you free from a life lived as a slave to the Chemical Religion's agenda. Hold on to these five simple steps. Put them into practice.

1. Hope Filled Mind
2. Tap Into God's Power Source
3. Get Back to the Garden
4. Breath in Energy

5.  Repent of Toxins

## Choose Life!

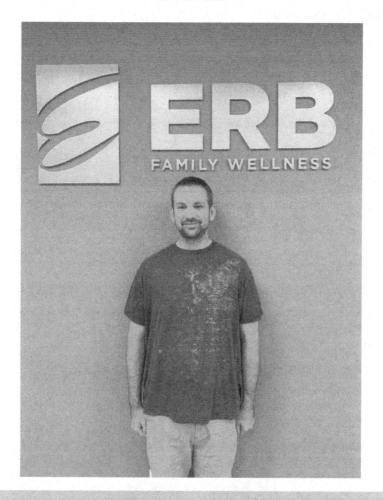

I started going to Erb Family Wellness because I slipped a disk in my back. I thought they were just regular chiropractors. Turns out they not only healed my back pain, but I noticed I wasn't having migraines anymore since the subluxation was being corrected. I had been having migraines several times a week for the ten years since I returned from Afghanistan. In less than ten weeks since beginning treatment, the Erbs did so much more than I had expected. They have taught me about nutrition, the dangers of sugar and the importance of spinal care. They are always providing educational classes to patients and the community. I just started treatment ten weeks ago. It has been a pretty quick turn-around. – Jason Nance

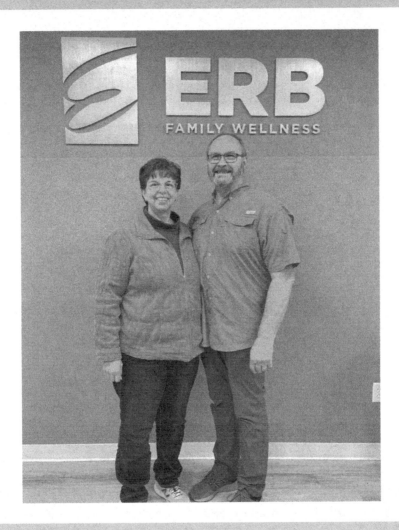

I've been unhealthy and very overweight my whole adult life. I came to Erb Family wellness with joint issues. Earlier in the year I had developed a lot of pain in my arms and shoulders. John and I had been looking for a chiropractor when I happened to go to lunch with a friend who is a

patient of the Erbs. She was telling me how wonderful the care was that she and her family received from them and invited me to a "Friends and Family" event to meet Dr.'s David and Kimberly. John was still skeptical, but they said we both needed to come in and, "since you're here John, we are going to look at you too." He believed in chiropractors, but it had been a long time since he was able to find a good one.

I started care on July 16, 2021, and John waited a week. He said I was going to be the guinea pig and go first. Since then, we have had a snowball of activity going on. We started listening to their teachings. It all made sense. They were saying all the right things about nutrition, mental health, spinal adjustments, avoiding toxins and exercise. We've been eating the most advanced diet plan since the 1st of August 2021 (for about three months.)

John was on blood pressure meds and was also taking meds for acid reflux that he had suffered from for 40 years. He was on an asthma/respiratory medication, and he took allergy meds twice a day.

It only took about a month of adjustments and sticking to the diet plan the Erbs recommended, and John is off all meds. He has lost 35 pounds! His medical doctor confirmed his blood pressure is way down. He's feeling so good that he has been able to go walking again. John's hip pain and blurred vision had been so bad that he had to give up walking before going to Erb Family Wellness.

As for me, I tried every diet at least once or 900 times before coming to Dr. Erb. If I lost any weight, it would be maybe four pounds. Bariatric surgery didn't even work. I lost about 25 pounds, but it came right back! I even went to a weight loss clinic and after three months I had only lost four pounds. The manager took me in the back and told me I needed mental help for paying all this money to lose weight but cheating. I wasn't cheating! But since I started with the Erbs I have lost 30 pounds. I've gone down two and a half sizes. I'm starting to get excited to wear some clothes styles that I haven't been able to wear since I was in my early 20's!

At some point in the last 40 years, we had tried everything. But the Erbs showed us how to put all five practices together at once to restore our health and help us to begin reaching our goals.

I'm still dealing with some pain, but I no longer take ibuprofen like I did before. I'm a work in progress, but I have hope again. I had nearly given up before finding Erb Family Wellness. They gave me hope and that is one of the biggest things they have restored to me. - John and Mary Reece

# APPENDIX

## What to Avoid List

**Cookware** made of aluminum and copper. When it is heated it leaches metal into the nutrition you eat. These trace metals are linked to Alzheimer's disease, cancers, hormone dysregulation, infertility, mental disorders, autoimmune disease, heart disease and the list goes on. I was shocked after having my own pans tested for toxicity, I discovered I was cooking up the potential for disease in the food I was feeding my family. Avoid these toxic cookware choices.

- Cast Iron
- Teflon
- Ceramic
- Stainless steels

**Microwaving.** Created by Nazis in WWII, microwaving kills 98% of cancer fighting nutrients in broccoli and the life energy nutrients in other foods, while creating carcinogenic substances in foods. Hans Hertel, a Swiss food scientist, initiated the first tests on microwaved food and microwave cooking to determine how microwaves affect human physiology and the blood. After studying these effects, Hertel concluded that microwaving food leads to food degeneration. These degenerative changes in nutrients caused changes in blood, which could cause health problems.

Health issues which could be caused from microwaving are:

- Elevated cholesterol levels.

- Plummeting white blood cells, which could suggest poisoning.

- Decreased red blood cell levels.

- Production of radiolytic compounds.

- Decreased hemoglobin levels, which might indicate anemia.

**Grilling** forms carcinogenic chemicals such as Heterocyclic amines (HCAs) and polycyclic aromatic hydrocarbons (PAHs).

**Canned Food/Plastics** contain BPA, a carcinogen shown to have negative health effects on the brain, behavior and prostate gland of fetuses, infants and children. It may also be linked to high blood pressure.

**Artificial Sweeteners** are linked to numerous cancers, including oral cavity and pharynx, colon, breast, ovarian, prostate and kidney. Some are linked to migraines, as they eat holes in the brain. Often defeating the purpose for which they are consumed, they are known to slow metabolism.

- Aspartame AKA AminoSweet - NutraSweet, Equal

- Acesulfame Potassium – Sunett, Sweet One

- Neotame - N/A

- Saccharin - Sweet 'N Low, Sweet Twin, Sugar Twin

- Sucralose – Splenda

**Pesticides & Herbicides** such as Roundup **have been** found on many food products on the shelves of grocery stores.

**Steroids are** found in many meats. They are used as a hormone to increase growth in livestock.

**Antibiotics are** found in many meats. They are used to ward off infection and illness in livestock.

**Mercury is** found in fish, some vaccines, old paint, dental fillings and can lead to cardiovascular risks, reproductive issues, and neurological damage.

**Ethanol,** found in alcohol, can cause liver cirrhosis, cancers, nervous system disorders and fetal alcohol syndrome are among the more serious pathologies.

**Sunset Yellow,** found in soft drinks to give them their red, yellow, or orange color. It's associated with behavioral issues in children.

**High Fructose Corn Syrup (HFCS) is** a hormone disruptor found in many packaged, processed, sugary foods and soft drinks. It is also linked to mercury toxicity.

**Hydrogenated Fats and Oils are** found in many packaged, processed foods can affect heart health because they increase "bad" (low-density lipoprotein, or LDL) cholesterol and lower "good" (high-density lipoprotein, or HDL) cholesterol.

**Arsenic is** found in rat poison, cigarettes and sometimes drinking water. It can cause skin cancer and cancers of the bladder and lungs.

**Triclosan is** found in anti-bacterial soaps. It interferes with the body's thyroid hormone metabolism and may be a potential endocrine disruptor. Children exposed to antibacterial compounds at an early age also have an increased chance of developing allergies, asthma and eczema.

**Phthalates is** found in water bottles, cosmetics, healthcare products and other items like soaps and toiletries. It can damage the liver, kidneys, lungs and reproductive system. They also increase feminization in males due to their xenotropic properties.

**Perchlorate is sometimes** found in water, tobacco or chemically treated solutions. It can cause low level thyroid activity.

**Perchloroethylene is** used as a dry-cleaning solvent. It has shown an association with several kinds of cancer according to the EPA's 2012 press release. They also warned of respiratory tract and eye irritation, kidney dysfunction and neurological effects.

**Dioxins are** found naturally in meats and fish and may result in skin lesions such as chloracne and patchy darkening of the skin, as well as altered liver function, impairment of the immune system, the developing nervous system, the endocrine system and reproductive functions.

**Lead is** found in some paint, in polluted soil and water and nearly everything made in China. It may cause anemia, weakness and kidney and brain damage, and even death. It can damage a developing baby's nervous system.

**Chlorine** in pool disinfectants and drinking water is associated with bladder, rectal and breast cancers. Chlorine heated in a hot shower or hot tub turns to gas and is linked to diseases of the lungs and tooth corrosion.

**Fluoride is used** in some toothpaste and used to treat water. It has been linked to several cancers, bone diseases, arthritis, cardiovascular and an array of other alarming diseases. It was also used by Nazi's in concentration camps to make the victims compliant.

**Cyanide is** found in some fruits, nuts, seeds and vegetables. It is linked to convulsions, loss of consciousness, low blood pressure, lung injury, respiratory failure leading to death and slow heart rate.

**Formaldehyde is** found in air fresheners, furniture, e-cigarettes and even some clothes. It can result in respiratory symptoms and eye, nose and throat irritation. Lung and nasopharyngeal cancer have also been associated with exposure.

**Parabens,** added to many deodorants, toothpastes, shampoos, conditioners, body lotions and makeups have been linked to increased risk of breast cancer and reproductive toxicity. Research demonstrates that parabens mimic estrogen and can trigger reactions such as increasing breast cell division and the growth of tumors.

**Copper is** found in copper cookware or drinking water. The metal can cause irritation of the nose, mouth and eyes and it causes headaches, stomachaches, dizziness, vomiting and diarrhea. It may cause liver and kidney damage and even death.

**EMFs** are electromagnetic field radiation. Subtle energies constantly swirl in and around our bodies, whether or not we are aware of them. EMFs are energy waves with frequencies below 300 hertz or cycles per second. The electromagnetic fields we encounter daily come from everyday things such as power lines, radar and microwave towers, television and computer screens, motors, fluorescent lights, microwave ovens, cell phones, electric blankets, house wiring and hundreds of other common electrical devices.

EMFs can cause cancer and unusual growths such as parotid tumors and brain tumors, along with a whole list of other alarming symptoms:

- Sleep disturbances, including insomnia
- Headache
- Depression and depressive symptoms
- Tiredness and fatigue
- Dysesthesia (a painful, often itchy sensation)
- Lack of concentration
- Changes in memory
- Dizziness
- Irritability
- Loss of appetite and weight loss
- Restlessness and anxiety
- Nausea
- Skin burning and tingling

https://erbfamilywellness.com

http://erbfamilydetox.com/customized-metabolix-testing/

http://erbfamilythermography.com

http://erbfamilyhyperbaric.com

Chemicalreligion.com

# END NOTES

**Chapter One:**

International Mortality Statistics (1981) by Michael Alderson

- Illich, I. *Medical Nemesis*. Chapter 1-The Epidemics of Modern Medicine, NY: Bantam Books 1976

- NVIC.org

- Kessler D. *JAMA*, 1993; 269 (No.21): 2785. Only about 1% of serious events are reported to the FDA

- Mendelsohn, R. *How To Raise A Healthy Child In Spite Of Your Doctor* Chicago: Contemporary Books 1984

- Dissolving Illusions Suzanne Humphries, MD; Roman Bystrianyk

- *American Association for Cancer Research*, San Francisco, CA. April 10, 2002. www.bmn.com_

- *Science* 1999; 286:1832.

- A Better Way movie

**Chapter Two:**

EWG July 14th 2005 Body Burden: The Pollution in Newborns

Hardick, B.J. (2018). *Align Your Health*. Celebration, FL:Maximized Living LP.

https://www.heart.org/en/healthy-living/healthy-eating/eat-smart/nutrition-basics/understanding-food-nutrition-labels

https://www.fix.com/blog/what-to-look-for-on-nutrition-labels/

https://www.nongmoproject.org/

https://www.mayoclinic.org/healthy-lifestyle/nutrition-and-healthy-eating/expert-answers/bpa/faq-20058331

https://www.ams.usda.gov/rules-regulations/organic/labeling

https://www.forthepeople.com/defective-product-lawyers/round-up-weed-killer-lawsuit/?utm_source=google&utm_medium=cpc&utm_campaign=6445831571&utm_device=c&utm_term=roundup%20and%20cancer&ads_cmpid=6445831571&ads_adid=78519509178&ads_matchtype=b&ads_network=g&ads_creative=377162923639&utm_term=roundup%20and%20cancer&ads_targetid=kwd-299448312638&utm_kxconfid=ty6howcay&g-clid=EAIaIQobChMIo4iCj-qa6gIVyEXVCh1jbgo2EAAYAiAAEgIvD_D_BwE

https://www.theguardian.com/lifeandstyle/2005/may/15/foodanddrink.shopping3

https://www.huffpost.com/entry/donald-rumsfeld-and-the-s_b_805581

https://www.aarda.org/gmo-foods-leaky-gut-inflammation/

https://www.reuters.com/article/gmcrops-safety/french-study-finds-tumours-in-rats-fed-gm-corn-idUSL5E8KJAGN20120919

https://naturalsociety.com/microwaves/#ixzz6XkjWXbUG

https://ehchiropractorlakemary.com/stop-the-madness-2/

https://www.mygenefood.com/blog/
why-glyphosate-is-dangerous-and-how-to-avoid-eating-it/

https://www.medicalnewstoday.com/articles/17685#sources

**Chapter Three:**

JPhysiol. 2010 Aug 1;588 (Pt15):2861-72. Epub 2010 Jun 14. Richards
JC, Johnson TK, Kuzma

https://www.niddk.nih.gov/health-information/diabetes/overview/
symptoms-causes

https://maxliving.com/healthy-articles/glucose-insulin-obesity-and-dia-
betes-type-2-whats-the-common-connection/

https://www.cdc.gov/media/releases/2017/p0718-diabetes-report.html

https://www.medicalnewstoday.com/articles/317246

https://jamanetwork.com/journals/jamainternalmedicine/
fullarticle/1819573

https://www.who.int/news-room/fact-sheets/detail/diabetes

https://sugarscience.ucsf.edu/hidden-in-plain-sight/#.X2EAQS05TjC

food pyramid https://www.center4research.org/
myplate-new-alternative-food-pyramid/

Diabetologia Journal

American Heart Association Meeting Report --Abstract 18838 (Hall
A2 --Poster T 2088)

https://www.youtube.com/watch?v=F6rTBW-dAB4_

**Chapter Four:**

Brain cholesterol Doctor David Pearlmutter M.D.

https://www.mayoclinic.org/diseases-conditions/heart-disease/symptoms-causes/syc-20353118

https://www.sciencedaily.com/releases/2015/05/150529193554.htm

https://maxliving.com/healthy-articles/back-pain-neck-pain-discovering-chiropractic-care-and-what-to-expect/

https://ehchiropractorlakemary.com/stop-the-madness-2/

The Pursuit of Health Dr. H.Gilbert Welch, Dr. Lisa M. Schwartz, and Dr. Steven Woloshin

Lucia Huff Pictured below

**Chapter Five:**

https://slate.com/human-interest/2013/02/where-do-the-millions-of-cancer-research-dollars-go-every-year.html

https://www.cancernetwork.com/view/costs-cancer-care-united-states-implications-action

https://www.nih.gov/news-events/news-releases/cancer-costs-projected-reach-least-158-billion-2020

https://www.cancer.gov/publications/dictionaries/cancer-terms/def/cancer

https://www.ncbi.nlm.nih.gov/pmc/articles/PMC2866629/

https://pdfs.semanticscholar.org/fed6/cb9108d6332ad1882da9f16ed-10d9a5cf5e3.pdf

http://www.scielo.br/scielo.php?pid=S1517-86922012000300015&script=sci_arttext&tlng=en

https://www.cancer.org/latest-news/exercise-linked-with-lower-risk-of-13-types-of-cancer.html

https://www.cancer.gov/about-cancer/causes-prevention/risk/obesity/physical-activity-fact-sheet

https://www.ncbi.nlm.nih.gov/pubmed/21461921

https://www.ncbi.nlm.nih.gov/pmc/articles/PMC2515569/

https://onlinelibrary.wiley.com/doi/epdf/10.3322/caac.21440

https://www.healthline.com/nutrition/why-refined-carbs-are-bad#section2

https://www.sciencedaily.com/releases/2016/04/160405182105.htm

https://www.youtube.com/watch?v=wY-JZ6TTNh8&feature=youtu.be

https://en.wikipedia.org/wiki/Otto_Heinrich_Warburg#Cancer_hypothesis

https://www.prnewswire.com/news-releases/otto-heinrich-warburg--the-free-radical-theory-an-abundant-supply-of-oxygen--antioxidants-for-disease-prevention-and-treatment-of-cancer-heart-attack-diabetes-and-other-diseases-259901311.html

https://www.cureyourowncancer.org/exposing-the-fraud-and-mythology-of-conventional-cancer-treatments.html

https://www.cureyourowncancer.org/exposed-deadly-cancer-drugs-make-cancer-worse-and-kill-patients-more-quickly.html

https://www.cureyourowncancer.org/study-accidentally-finds-chemo-makes-cancer-worse.html

https://livelovefruit.com/chemotherapy-kills/

https://journals.plos.org/plosone/article?id=10.1371/journal.
pone.0098246

https://rethinkingcancer.org/resources/cancer-forum/8_11-12/
the-untreated-live-longer/

https://www.medscape.com/viewarticle/893178

https://www.ajmc.com/view/variation-in-markups-on-outpatient-oncolo-gy-services-in-the-united-states

https://www.drkarafitzgerald.com/2016/08/02/episode-16-cancer-mito-chondrial-metabolic-disease-calorie-restricted-ketogenic-diet/

https://storemytumor.com/services/chemo-sensitivity-testing/

https://www.chrisbeatcancer.com/the-business-of-chemo/

Kent, Christopher. Models of Vertebral Subluxation: A Review. Journal of Vertebral Subluxation Research. August 1996, Vol 1:1. Pg. 4-5

Sternberg EM, Chrousos GP, Wilder RL, Gold PW. The stress response and the regulation of inflammatory disease. Ann Intern Med 1992; 117 (10):854

Brennan PC, Triano JJ, McGregor M, et al. Enhanced neutrophil respiratory burst as a biological marker for manipulation forces: duration of the effect and association with substance P and tumor necrosis factor. J Manipulative Physiol Ther 1992; 15(2):83

**Chapter Six:**

https://blog.weatherops.com/why-do-hurricanes-go-where-they-go

https://www.nssl.noaa.gov/education/svrwx101/thunderstorms/

http://www.rense.com/general34/quotes.htm

https://www.defendershield.com/
emf-immune-system-affects-disease-chronic-illness

https://www.greenmedinfo.com/disease/rheumatoid-arthritis

http://www.renegadetribune.com/
emfs-linked-to-cancer-autoimmunity-immune-dysfunction/

Department of Biophysics, Kobe University Graduate School of Health
Science, Kobe, Japan

NVIC.org

https://rense.com/general34/quotes.htm

**Chapter Seven:**

Caroline Leaf https://drleaf.com/blogs/news/
the-chemical-imbalance-myth?_pos=1&_sid=31319ab58&_ss=r

https://www.madinamerica.com/2018/06/
rising-rates-suicide-acknowledge-something-isnt-working/

https://www.psychologytoday.com/us/blog/side-effects/201008/
big-pharmas-role-in-promoting-dsm-disorders

https://www.ncbi.nlm.nih.gov/books/NBK217810/

https://spinalresearch.com.au/stress-brain-body-connection/ https://
www.ncbi.nlm.nih.gov/books/NBK10877/

https://www.verywellmind.com/the-anatomy-of-the-brain-2794895

https://adc.bmj.com/content/89/3/244

https://hms.harvard.edu/sites/default/files/assets/OCER/files/Taking%20
It%20All%20In%20Reading%20Materials%20Web.pdf

https://www.washingtonpost.com/news/to-your-health/wp/2018/06/07/u-s-suicide-rates-rise-sharply-across-the-country-new-report-shows/?noredirect=on

**https://www.themindfulnessclinic.ca/high-intensity-interval-training-hiit-for-anxiety-depression-and-fitness/**

https://www.youtube.com/watch?v=dw_4hTK1_ek

**https://www.mayoclinic.org/healthy-lifestyle/stress-management/in-depth/exercise-and-stress/art-20044469**

Gunnars, K. (2015, April 15). "20 Foods That Are Bad For Your Health (Avoid Them!)." Healthline. Retrieved from https://www.healthline.com/nutrition/20-foods-to-avoid-like-the-plague

Hardick, B.J. (2018). *Align Your Health*. Celebration, FL:Maximized Living LP.

Dean, A.,& Armstrong, J. (2009, May 8). "Genetically Modified Foods." *American Academy of Environmental Medicine*. Retrieved from https://www.aaemonline.org/gmo.php

"Frequently asked questions on genetically modified foods." (2014, May). World Health Organization. Retrieved from http://www.who.int/foodsafety/areas_work/food-technology/faq-genetically-modified-food/en/

https://www.nrdc.org/stories/mercury-guide

https://www.mindbodygreen.com/0-14560/10-reasons-why-stress-is-the-most-dangerous-toxin-in-your-life.html

https://www.epa.gov/air-trends/particulate-matter-pm25-trends

https://www.sleepfoundation.org/articles/how-much-sleep-do-we-really-need

Psychiatric Drug Withdrawal – Peter R. Breggin

Confessions from a Pharmaceutical Pusher – Gwen Olsen

https://www.psychiatrictimes.com/view/
movement-disturbances-associated-ssris

https://www.ncbi.nlm.nih.gov/pmc/articles/PMC3726098/

https://www.ncbi.nlm.nih.gov/pmc/articles/PMC3325428/

https://constantinereport.com/
eli-lilly-ghostwrote-articles-to-market-zyprexa-files-show/

https://www.britannica.com/science/thalamus

Wamsley, et al., 1987

Malberg, Eisch, Nestler & Duman, 2000

Andrews, Kornstein, Halberstadt, Gardner and Neale

Minnesota Community Measurement 2010

Ljung, Bjorkenstam, and Bjorkenstam, 2008

Sundell, 2011

## Chapter Eight:

https://www.medicalnewstoday.com/articles/
accutane-side-effects#side-effects

https://cycleharmony.com/remedies/hormone-imbalance/
top-10-xenoestrogens-the-primary-cause-of-estrogen-dominance

https://www.ncbi.nlm.nih.gov/pmc/articles/PMC5051569/

https://www.dailymail.co.uk/health/article-1388888/GM-food-toxins-
blood-93-unborn-babies.html

https://www.huffpost.com/entry/monsanto-roundup-ready-miscarriages-n_827135?guccounter=1&guce_referrer=aHR0cHM6Ly90b2RheX-NtYW1hLmNvbS9wcmVnbmFuY3ktYmlydGGgvZ21vcy1taXNjYX-JyaWFnZS1pbmZlcnRpbGl0eS1wcmVtV0ZXJtLWxhYm9yLWFuZ-C1iaXJ0aC1kZWZlY3Rz&guce_referrer_sig=AQAAAJ9Y-YuwvJ9b4T-VW6thgA6FnnTc3T0jEXW0savNkB8jyxj3MHTN28WOTzmMXP-1Dim4ZSbOFXEr3jArNKMBXZw20vk6deRYg_hcZ4f_ugy0Q2Z6fHs-1kzEsdBI_Z7mG77SYsyR8_goBxQ4qdi29wGLm6wbT98jAckIkbZm-w6SGHpg

https://www.gmwatch.org/en/news/latest-news/18245-argen-tine-study-links-glyphosate-herbicide-to-miscarriage-birth-defects

https://www.mayoclinic.org/diseases-conditions/pregnancy-loss-miscarriage/symptoms-causes/syc-20354298

https://www.sands.org.au/miscarriage

https://www.sciencealert.com/meta-analysis-finds-majority-of-hu-man-pregnancies-end-in-miscarriage-biorxiv

https://todaysmama.com/pregnancy-birth/gmos-miscarriage-infertility-preterm-labor-and-birth-defects

https://www.gmoscience.org/pesticides-in-foods-can-harm-human-fertility/

https://www.scirp.org/Journal/PaperInformation.aspx?PaperID=83267

https://www.ewg.org/enviroblog/2008/02/future-generations-face-rising-infertility-rates

https://www.scientificamerican.com/article/rats-harmed-by-great-grandmothers-exposure-to-dioxin/

https://pubmed.ncbi.nlm.nih.gov/20955784/

https://www.ewg.org/enviroblog/2017/03/swimming-upstream-against-infertility-what-you-can-do-protect-your-sperm

https://www.drugs.com/inactive/polysorbate-80-372.html

https://pubmed.ncbi.nlm.nih.gov/8473002/

https://www.westonaprice.org/health-topics/vaccinations/adjuvants-in-vaccines/

https://www.ovarian-cysts-pcos.com/pcos-roundup.html

https://truthsnitch.com/tag/polysorbate-80-linked-to-infertility/#sthash.gIzUKVNH.OblstBh8.dpbs

https://en.wikipedia.org/wiki/Bacillus_thuringiensis

https://www.hormone.org/your-health-and-hormones/endocrine-disrupting-chemicals-edcs

https://www.drugwatch.com/yaz/lawsuits/

https://www.chicagotribune.com/lifestyles/health/ct-met-birth-control-risks-20130915-story.html

https://pubmed.ncbi.nlm.nih.gov/27680324/

https://pubmed.ncbi.nlm.nih.gov/30193687/

https://www.aafp.org/afp/2006/1201/p1915.html#afp20061201p1915-b1

https://www.aafp.org/afp/2006/1201/p1915.html

https://www.drugwatch.com/manufacturers/bayer/

https://www.chicagotribune.com/lifestyles/health/ct-met-birth-control-risks-20130915-story.html

https://www.drugs.com/sfx/accutane-side-effects.html

https://www.foxnews.com/story/
study-says-accutane-worse-for-heart-liver-than-thought

https://www.ncbi.nlm.nih.gov/pmc/articles/PMC4528880/

https://en.wikipedia.org/wiki/Human_papillomavirus_infection

https://www.healthline.com/health/pregnancy/how-does-clomid-work

https://www.drugs.com/sfx/clomid-side-effects.html

https://pubmed.ncbi.nlm.nih.gov/28547654/

https://www.nhs.uk/medicines/metformin/

https://www.verywellfamily.com/
treatment-with-metformin-for-pcos-and-infertility-1960178#citation-5

https://www.schmidtlaw.com/metformin-class-action-lawsuit/

https://www.forbes.com/sites/learnvest/2014/02/06/the-cost-of-ivf-4-
things-i-learned-while-battling-infertility/#4113de9a24dd

https://pubmed.ncbi.nlm.nih.gov/15665017/

https://pubmed.ncbi.nlm.nih.gov/26296545/

https://www.hli.org/resources/products-that-use-aborted-fetuses/

https://www.medicalnewstoday.com/articles/17685#types

https://www.who.int/en/news-room/fact-sheets/detail/
dioxins-and-their-effects-on-human-health

https://www.ncbi.nlm.nih.gov/pmc/articles/PMC5080866/#B7

https://www.womenshealth.gov/a-z-topics/emergency-contraception
https://embryo.asu.edu/pages/diethylstilbestrol-des-us

**Chapter Nine:**

**https://www.thehealthyhomeeconomist.**
**com/50-in-utero-human-studies-confirm-risks-prenatal-ultrasound/**

https://www.drugs.com/mtm/pitocin.html

https://sarahbuckley.com/
epidurals-risks-and-concerns-for-mother-and-baby/

https://www.worldometers.info/abortions/

https://www.biblegateway.com/
passage/?search=Psalm+139&version=NIV

https://www.fda.gov/consumers/consumer-updates/
avoid-fetal-keepsake-images-heartbeat-monitors

https://www.thehealthyhomeeconomist.
com/50-in-utero-human-studies-confirm-risks-prenatal-ultrasound/

https://www.amazon.com/gp/product/1941719023/ref=as_li_
qf_sp_asin_il_tl?ie=UTF8&camp=1789&creative=9325&cre-
ativeASIN=1941719023&linkCode=as2&tag=theheahomec0a-20&link-
Id=TXCNSCTUNRAYG2ML

https://www.whattoexpect.com/wom/pregnancy/0723/is-your-doctor-or-
dering-too-many-ultrasounds-.aspx

https://biblehub.com/proverbs/31-8.htm

World Health Organization, Care in Normal Birth: A Practical
Guide. Report of a Technical Working Group (Geneva: World Health
Organization, 1996): 16

https://www.washingtonpost.com/national/health-science/the-big-num-
ber--21-percent-of-babies-are-born-by-c-section-nearly-double-the-
rate-in-2000/2018/11/16/ae539bfe-e8ef-11e8-bbdb-72fdbf9d4fed_story.
html

https://www.thecut.com/2018/12/how-much-does-it-actually-cost-to-give-birth.html

https://my.clevelandclinic.org/health/articles/15274-the-benefits-of-breastfeeding-for-baby--for-mom

https://www.tandfonline.com/doi/abs/10.1080/19440049.2017.1419286?journalCode=tfac20

McKeever TM, Lewis SA, Smith C. Does vaccination increase the risk of developing allergic disease?: A birth cohort study. Winter Abstract supplement to *Thorax*, 2002; 57: Supplement III

*From Childhood Vaccination – Questions all parents should ask* (p. 22)

(Cherry et al. *Pediatrics Supplement.* 1988;973).

https://www.momsadvocatingsustainability.org/gmos-in-baby-formula-what/

https://www.momsacrossamerica.com/monsanto_s_roundup_found_in_baby_food

https://journals.sagepub.com/doi/full/10.1177/2050312120925344

https://www.gingerblossomdoula.com/post/why-would-a-baby-or-child-see-a-chiropractor

https://www.todaysparent.com/baby/breastfeeding/magical-ways-breastmilk-changes-to-meet-your-babys-needs/

https://milkgenomics.org/article/protective-cells-in-breast-milk-for-the-infant-and-the-mother/

Odent ME, Culpin EE, Kimmel T, Pertussis vaccination and asthma: is there a link? Letter. *JAMA.* 1994; 272(8):593

Coulter HL. *Vaccination, Social Violence and Criminality: The Medical Assault on the American Brain.* Washington, DC: Center for Empirical Medicine. 1990

*Epidemiology,* 1997;8:678-680. Note: comparison of DPT and non-DPT children

*When Your Doctor Is Wrong: Hepatitis B Vaccine & Autism* by Judy Converse, MPH, RD [Xlibris Corporation]

Coulter HL. *Vaccination, Social Violence and Criminality: The Medical Assault on the American Brain.* Washington, DC: Center for Empirical Medicine. 1990

(Anne Murray, et al.)

Carol Sepkoski et al.

https://www.cesareanrates.org

Odent ME, Culpin EE, Kimmel T, Pertussis vaccination and asthma: is there a link? Letter. *JAMA.* 1994; 272(8):593

9Mawson, *et al.*0.

(McKeever TM, Lewis SA, Smith C. Does vaccination increase the risk of developing allergic disease?: A birth cohort study. Winter Abstract supplement to *Thorax,* 2002; 57: Supplement III)

*Morbidity and Mortality Weekly Report.* US Govt. 6/6/86/35(22):366-70

(*Mothering Magazine.* May/June 1999).

(The role of vaccines in arthritis and autoimmunity – 'vaccinosis': a dangerous liaison? *J Autoimmune* 2000;14(1):1-10)

Illich, I. *Medical Nemesis.* Chapter 1-The Epidemics of Modern Medicine, NY: Bantam Books 1976

Coulter HL. *Vaccination, Social Violence and Criminality: The Medical Assault on the American Brain*. Washington, DC: Center for Empirical Medicine. 1990.

**Chapter Ten:**

https://www.medicalnewstoday.com/articles/
accutane-side-effects#side-effects

https://www.drugs.com/sfx/accutane-side-effects.html

https://www.foxnews.com/story/
study-says-accutane-worse-for-heart-liver-than-thought

https://www.honeycolony.com/article/accutane-cancer-acne/

https://www.ncbi.nlm.nih.gov/pmc/articles/PMC3726098/

https://www.todaysparent.com/baby/breastfeeding/
magical-ways-breastmilk-changes-to-meet-your-babys-needs/

https://www.researchgate.net/
publication/261370424_Diethylstilbestrol_Story

https://americanaddictioncenters.org/adderall/mixing-with-alcohol

https://americanaddictioncenters.org/adderall/
adderall-abuse-among-college-students

https://www.jhsph.edu/news/news-releases/2016/adderall-misuse-rising-
among-young-adults.html

https://www.consumeraffairs.com/news/energy-drinks-the-cause-of-
many-sudden-cardiac-deaths-in-young-people-researchers-find-040315.
html

https://www.forthepeople.com/defective-product-lawyers/
monster-energy-drinks-lawsuit/

https://www.schmidtandclark.com/xanax-lawsuit

https://www.verywellmind.com/benzodiazepine-withdrawal-4588452

https://www.hopkinsmedicine.org/health/wellness-and-prevention/
what-does-vaping-do-to-your-lungs

https://vertavahealth.com/polysubstances/xanax-adderall/

https://www.hhs.gov/opioids/about-the-epidemic/index.html

https://www.propublica.org/article/
senate-panel-investigates-drug-company-ties-to-pain-groups

https://www.forbes.com/sites/quora/2019/11/07/what-role-did-doctors-
and-drug-companies-play-in-the-opioid-crisis/?sh=6e7e4a93612d

https://www.drugabuse.gov/drug-topics/trends-statistics/
overdose-death-rates

https://www.who.int/news-room/fact-sheets/detail/opioid-overdose

https://public3.pagefreezer.com/browse/HHS.gov/31-12-2020T08:51/
https://www.hhs.gov/about/news/2017/10/26/hhs-acting-secretary-de-
clares-public-health-emergency-address-national-opioid-crisis.html

https://www.drugs.com/sfx/accutane-side-effects.html

https://www.foxnews.com/story/
study-says-accutane-worse-for-heart-liver-than-thought

https://www.honeycolony.com/article/accutane-cancer-acne/

https://www.theguardian.com/society/2019/dec/27/
suicides-linked-to-acne-drug-roaccutane-as-regulator-reopens-inquiry

https://www.betterhealth.vic.gov.au/health/healthyliving/
the-dangers-of-sitting?viewAsPdf=true

https://www.dailykos.com/stories/2015/5/26/1387827/-DEA-approves-first-drug-trial-of-ecstasy-to-treat-anxiety-and-depression

https://projects.propublica.org/graphics/bigpharma

https://www.saunderslawyers.com/top-eight-largest-drug-lawsuit-settlements-time/

https://www.huffpost.com/entry/holding-big-pharma-accoun_b_8280952

https://www.nytimes.com/2015/09/20/health/fda-nominee-califfs-ties-to-drug-industry-raise-questions.html?_r=0

https://www.dailysignal.com/2020/09/29/covid-19-linked-to-rising-suicide-rates-among-teens/

https://www.cnn.com/2019/10/29/health/common-sense-kids-media-use-report-wellness/index.html

https://www.hrsa.gov/enews/past-issues/2019/january-17/loneliness-epidemic

https://www.hrsa.gov/enews/past-issues/2019/january-17/loneliness-epidemic

**https://www.ncbi.nlm.nih.gov/pmc/articles/PMC3255175/**

https://www.heart.org/en/healthy-living/healthy-lifestyle/quit-smoking-tobacco/is-vaping-safer-than-smoking

https://www.yalemedicine.org/conditions/evali

https://www.webmd.com/lung/popcorn-lung#2

https://www.cdc.gov/tobacco/basic_information/e-cigarettes/severe-lung-disease.html#what-we-know

https://rense.com/general34/quotes.htm

*Journal of American Medical Association*

## Chapter Eleven:

https://www.americashealthrankings.org/explore/annual/measure/Sedentary/state/ALL

https://www.health.harvard.edu/mind-and-mood/why-behavior-change-is-hard-and-why-you-should-keep-trying

https://www.ncbi.nlm.nih.gov/pmc/articles/PMC3207358/#R12

https://www.ncbi.nlm.nih.gov/pmc/articles/PMC4626078/

https://www.cancer.gov/about-cancer/understanding/statisticshttps://www.cancer.gov/about-cancer/understanding/statistics

https://www.ncbi.nlm.nih.gov/pubmed/20935133/

https://www.ncbi.nlm.nih.gov/pmc/articles/PMC3726719/

https://www.dovepress.com/the-western-diet-and-lifestyle-and-diseases-of-civilization-peer-reviewed-article-RRCC

https://www.who.int/cancer/prevention/en/

http://www.aicr.org/cancer-research-update/2018/2-7/new-study-clarifies-how-alcohol-causes-cancer.html

https://www.cancer.org/cancer/cancer-causes/diet-physical-activity/alcohol-use-and-cancer.html

https://www.cancer.net/blog/podcasts/alcohol-and-cancer-with-noelle-k-loconte-md

https://www.ncbi.nlm.nih.gov/pubmed/7979220/

https://www.sciencedaily.com/releases/2007/09/070910132848.htm

https://www.ncbi.nlm.nih.gov/pubmed/19595811/

https://www.ncbi.nlm.nih.gov/pubmed/15974909/

https://www.peta.org/about-peta/faq/my-doctor-wants-me-to-take-pre-marin-but-i-understand-its-made-from-horse-urine-is-this-true/

https://www.nationalconsumerlawyers.com/hrt/lawsuit/

https://consumer.healthday.com/senior-citizen-information-31/senior-citizen-news-778/u-s-seniors-struggle-more-to-pay-for-health-care-compared-to-other-countries-728558.html

https://www.tendonitisexpert.com/medications-that-cause-osteoporosis.html

https://www.cdc.gov/vaccinesafety/concerns/thimerosal/index.html

https://pubmed.ncbi.nlm.nih.gov/16240488/

https://pubmed.ncbi.nlm.nih.gov/30664867/

https://content.iospress.com/articles/journal-of-alzheimers-disease/jad191140

Broyles, K. (2000). *The silenced voice speaks out: A study of abuse and neglect of nursing home residents.* Atlanta, GA: A report from the Atlanta Long Term Care Ombudsman Program and Atlanta Legal Aid Society to the National Citizens Coalition for Nursing Home Reform.

https://chappellhealth.com/2013/12/dr-fudenberg-on-flu-shots-alzheimers/

https://link.springer.com/chapter/10.1007/978-3-319-73820-8_13#CR96

Wells, Y., Foreman, P., Gething, L., & Petralia, W. (2004). Nurses' attitudes toward aging and older adults--examining attitudes and practices among health services providers in Australia. *Journal of Gerontological Nursing, 30*(9), 5–13.

Hayes, L. J., Orchard, C. A., McGillis Hall, L., Nincic, V., O'Brien-Pallas, L., & Andrews, G. (2006). Career intentions of nursing students and new nurse graduates: A review of the literature. *International Journal of Nursing Education Scholarship, 3*(1), Article26.

Ben-Harush, A., Shiovitz-Ezra, S., Doron, I., Alon, S., Leibovitz, A., Golander, H., et al. (2016). Ageism among physicians, nurses, and social workers: Findings from a qualitative study. *European Journal of Ageing, 14*, 39. https://doi.org/10.1007/s10433-016-0389-9

Boult, C., Boult, L. B., Morishita, L., Dowd, B., Kane, R. L., & Urdangarin, C. F. (2001). A randomized clinical trial of outpatient geriatric evaluation and management. *Journal of the American Geriatrics Society, 49*(4), 351–359.

Ambady, N. (2002). Physical therapists' nonverbal communication predicts geriatric patients' health outcomes. *Psychology and Aging, 17*(3), 443.

Greene, M. D., Adelman, R. D., & Rizzo, C. (1996). Problems in communication between physicians and older patients. *Journal of Geriatric Psychiatry, 29*(1), 13–32.

McLaughlin, T. J., Soumerai, S. B., Willison, D. J., Gurwitz, J. H., Borbas, C., Guadagnoli, E., et al. (1996). Adherence to national guidelines for drug treatment of suspected acute myocardial infarction: Evidence for undertreatment in women and the elderly. *Archives of Internal Medicine, 156*(7), 799–805.

https://oig.hhs.gov/oei/reports/oei-02-17-00020.asp

https://www.medicaresupplement.com/media/1029/true-link-report-on-elder-financial-abuse-012815.pdf

https://all.org/u-s-government-report-shows-hospice-abuse-sacrificing-patient-care-for-profit/

https://hospicekills.blogspot.com/2007/09/how-do-we-not-know.html

https://www.ncbi.nlm.nih.gov/pmc/articles/PMC534658/

http://www.apa.org/research/action/immune.aspx

*CareMore Health* https://www.hrsa.gov/enews/past-issues/2019/
january-17/loneliness-epidemic

https://www.biznews.com/thought-leaders/2020/12/16/retire-at-55-and-
live-to-80-work-till-youre-65-and-die-at-67-startling-new-data-shows-
how-work-pounds-older-bodies

https://www.apa.org/research/action/immune

https://www.cdc.gov/reproductivehealth/data_stats/#Hysterectomy

https://en.wikipedia.org/wiki/Hysteria

https://www.ajmc.com/view/
trends-in-mortality-following-hip-fracture-in-older-women

https://www.everydayhealth.com/news/
things-your-doctor-wont-tell-you-about-hysterectomy/

https://www.womenshealthmag.com/health/a34574411/
hysterectomy-side-effects/

https://www.heatherhirschmd.com

https://www.ncbi.nlm.nih.gov/pmc/articles/PMC4286861/

https://www.ncbi.nlm.nih.gov/pmc/articles/PMC5898981/

https://www.nytimes.com/2019/11/11/us/javaid-perwaiz-hysterecto-
mies-fallopian-tubes.html

https://www.uclahealth.org/christopher-tarnay

https://www.healthcentral.com/article/
the-link-between-a-hysterectomy-and-your-thyroid

https://academic.oup.com/jcem/article/101/10/3812/2764945

https://www.thegatewaypundit.com/2021/03/british-government-study-
confirms-covid-19-vaccine-risk-infections-increase-fortnight-jab/

https://defending-gibraltar.net/t/urgent-warning-on-covid-19-vaccine-re-
lated-deaths-in-the-elderly-and-care-homes/1230

https://www.womenshealth.gov/publications/our-publications/fact-sheet/
endometriosis.html

(above page removed??)

Lyanne McGuire, PhD, of John Hopkins School of Medicine with Kiecolt-
Glaser and Glaser, 2002.

Suzanne Segerstrom, PhD, of the University of Kentucky, and Gregory
Miller, PhD, of the University of British Columbia.

Valenstein et al., 2009

Wells et al. 2004

Hayes et al. 2006

McLaughlin et al. 1996

*Facts, Views and Vision: Issues in Obstetrics, Gynecology and
Reproductive Health*

(Broyles, 2000)

A study published in the *American Journal of Obstetrics & Gynecology*.

**Chapter Twelve:**

https://www.msn.com/en-gb/news/uknews/care-home-deaths-from-
covid-19-surge-to-highest-proportion-%20since-start-of-pandemic/
ar-BB1dkxTs

GAVI.org June 23, 2009

http://whale.to/vaccine/WHO2.pdf

WHO, Coronavirus disease (COVID-19): Serology June 9, 2020, What Is Herd Immunity section

WHO, Coronavirus disease (COVID-19): Herd immunity, lockdowns and COVID-19, October 2020 (Archived)

WHO, Coronavirus disease (COVID-19): Herd immunity, lockdowns and COVID-19, December 31, 2020

https://www.cuimc.columbia.edu/news/
anthony-fauci-discusses-covid-19-challenges-columbia-virologist

https://articles.mercola.com/sites/articles/archive/2021/03/19/
un-food-systems-summit-2021.aspx?ui=900c3f-
54d0a222e4de3e7896cb6d8f3d1733a83a920bbdf65970db72d3674e80&s-
d=20111010&cid_source=dnl&cid_medium=email&cid_content=ar-
t2ReadMore&cid=20210319_HL2&mid=DM833992&rid=1110804299

https://articles.mercola.com/sites/articles/archive/2021/03/19/
gavi-bill-gates-world-health-organization.aspx?ui=900c3f-
54d0a222e4de3e7896cb6d8f3d1733a83a920bbdf65970db72d3674e80&s-
d=20111010&cid_source=dnl&cid_medium=email&cid_content=art1H-
L&cid=20210319_HL2&mid=DM833992&rid=1110804299

https://www.usatoday.com/story/news/factcheck/2020/04/24/fact-
check-medicare-hospitals-paid-more-covid-19-patients-coronavi-
rus/3000638001/

https://open.lib.umn.edu/humanbiology/chapter/2-7-adaptive-immunity/

**https://youtu.be/SXO9GgfWvaQ**

https://erbfamilywellness-my.sharepoint.com/:p:/p/derb/Ed-

vHxq9OxttNmoevjT8UMUEBJ0jv77W4Ubp12GYm0GDcgQ-
?e=M2AwRv

https://www.theepochtimes.com/dr-robert-malone-mrna-vaccine-inven-tor-on-the-bioethics-of-experimental-vaccines-and-the-ultimate-gas-lighting_3889805.html

https://www.youtube.com/watch?v=swi0fQE_
RC4&fbclid=IwAR1AkKNUE4ZuLBHOSDKeGIzEt5m_wFjnXG8B-cjw-wtLi_2plkFjHbKdRfRs

https://www.cdc.gov/mmwr/volumes/70/wr/pdfs/mm7007e1-H.pdf

https://www.businessinsider.com/americans-dont-need-masks-penc
e-says-as-demand-increases-2020-2?fbclid=IwAR0WOZsYq36tuJ7l-HlMOwQe45z2T5aTBC-dzLyBSRD9aiQva1WdVJpRsFDo

https://www.who.int/publications-detail/advice-on-the-use-of-masks-in-the-community-during-home-care-and-in-healthcare-settings-in-the-context-of-the-novel-coronavirus-(2019-ncov)-outbreak
https://jamanetwork.com/journals/jama/fullarticle/2762694?fb-clid=IwAR1lVVfr4DbSZSydl5PZJA-mNjLM1sHVQqRrmxFGX14X-sctxY-cUqRgeJdQ

https://www.youtube.com/watch?v=PRa6t_e7dgI&feature=youtu.be&fb-clid=IwAR0K_ZRgZ9cssZA98NwPEGOjwhZRRsNFUPpS_zY6O3bJD-wO5SKkdW3o8GS0
https://www.acpjournals.org/doi/10.7326/M20-1342?fbclid=IwAR3Owp
QyY7NOnhyXyX0A2NUJUktLeLNH3NQMQ7qKBcvnl1guEX2C1jmm
VXY

https://video.foxnews.com/v/6137596907001#sp=show-clips

https://www.hsgac.senate.gov/imo/media/doc/Testimony-Ioannidis-2020-05-06.pdf (1918 flu)

The Case Against Masks Dr. Judy A. Mikovits, Kent Heckenlively, JD

<u>Corona False Alarm? Facts and Figures</u> Dr. Karina Reiss, Dr. Sucharit Bhakdi

https://www.technocracy.news/
blaylock-face-masks-pose-serious-risks-to-the-healthy/

https://www.pleasantfamilydentistry.com/blog/
what-is-mask-mouth-and-how-you-can-you-prevent-it

https://www.google.com/amp/s/sheerahministries.
com/2019/07/03/hebrew-year-5780-2020-a-year-
to-widen-your-mouth-in-wisdom-or-zip-it-shut/
amp/

https://podcasts.apple.com/us/podcast/
bret-weinstein-darkhorse-podcast/id1471581521?i=1000525032595

https://www.washingtonpost.com/national/health-science/triclosan-
found-in-antibacterial-soap-and-other-products-causes-cancer-in-
mice/2014/11/24/096b8ca4-70cc-11e4-ad12-3734c461eab6_story.html

https://draxe.com/health/fda-bans-triclosan/

https://www.ncbi.nlm.nih.gov/pmc/articles/PMC3983973/

https://mightynest.com/learn/research-by-concern/dangers-of-triclosan

https://www.disclose.tv/t/all-vaccinated-people-will-die-within-2-years-
nobel-laureate-luc-montagnier/32675

https://articles.mercola.com/sites/articles/archive/2021/03/19/
gavi-bill-gates-world-health-organization.aspx?ui=900c3f-
54d0a222e4de3e7896cb6d8f3d1733a83a920bbdf65970db72d3674e80&s-
d=20111010&cid_source=dnl&cid_medium=email&cid_content=ar-
t1ReadMore&cid=20210319_HL2&mid=DM833992&rid=1110804299

https://www.lifesitenews.com/opinion/
abp-vigano-on-truth-over-fear-covid-19-the-vaccine-and-the-great-reset

https://www.thegatewaypundit.com/2021/07/vaers-website-currently-of-fline-number-covid-vaccine-deaths-reaches-11405-listed-website/

https://www.americanthinker.com/articles/2021/03/covid_and_the_sem-melweis_reflex.html

https://www.youtube.com/watch?v=PyA_FlPCWUA

https://www.insurancejournal.com/news/national/2020/08/14/579150.htm

https://www.nbcnews.com/news/us-news/coronavirus-spreads-new-york-nursing-home-forced-take-recovering-patients-n1191811

https://www.americanthinker.com/blog/2021/03/covid_death_data_fraud.html

https://www.healthline.com/health/hugging-benefits#3.-Hugs-may-boost-your-heart-health

https://fee.org/articles/a-years-worth-of-suicide-attempts-in-four-weeks-the-unintended-consequences-of-covid-19-lockdowns/

https://news.yahoo.com/coronavirus-forces-100k-ny-small-192934579.html?soc_src=community&soc_trk=fb

https://heart.bmj.com/content/102/13/1009

https://journals.plos.org/plosmedicine/article/info%3A-doi%2F10.1371%2Fjournal.pmed.1000316

https://www.hrsa.gov/enews/past-issues/2019/january-17/loneliness-epidemic

https://jamanetwork.com/journals/jamapediatrics/fullarticle/205331

https://www.npr.org/2020/09/11/908773533/hangover-from-alcohol-boom-could-last-long-after-pandemic-ends

https://www.wsj.com/articles/more-people-are-taking-drugs-for-anxiety-and-insomnia-and-doctors-are-worried-11590411600

https://www.rcreader.com/commentary/questioning-unreliable-pcr-testing-is-hardly-trivial

**https://www.youtube.com/watch?v=a_Vy6fgaBPE**

https://www.scientificamerican.com/article/infant-touch/

https://katrinah.com/nutrition-protocol-to-neutralize-graphene-oxide/

https://ambassadorlove.wordpress.com/2021/08/09/confirmed-graphene-oxide-main-ingredient-in-covid-shots/

https://www.ncbi.nlm.nih.gov/pmc/articles/PMC6110298/

https://cairnsnews.org/2021/08/27/lying-fact-checkers-caught-out-on-not-so-secret-pfizer-moderna-contaminant/

https://www.humorousmathematics.com/post/the-adverse-effects-of-experimental-messenger-rna-mrna-vaccines-a-k-a-injections-for-covid-19

https://www.gettyimages.com/detail/news-photo/dr-arnold-monto-chair-of-vaccines-and-related-biological-news-photo/1230049191

https://www.lifesitenews.com/opinion/abp-vigano-on-truth-over-fear-covid-19-the-vaccine-and-the-great-reset

https://forbiddenknowledgetv.net/former-pfizer-employee-confirms-poison-in-covid-vaccine/

https://abcnews.go.com/Business/wireStory/pfizer-raises-2021-outlook-strong-q2-revenue-profit-79112896

https://www.bitchute.com/video/nCJgZLroYJiK/

https://beckernews.com/new-evidence-suggests-covid-vaccine-may-spread-the-virus-nbc-news-report-deleted-from-usa-today-article-40546/

https://www.americanthinker.com/blog/2021/06/vaccine_resisters_are_proving_hard_to_convince.html

https://web.archive.org/web/20201223100930/https:/www.who.int/emergencies/diseases/novel-corona-virus-2019/question-and-answers-hub/q-a-detail/herd-immunity-lockdowns-and-covid-19

https://afinalwarning.com/535134.html

http://bit.ly/GertV

(above removed)

https://afinalwarning.com/535134.html

https://my.clevelandclinic.org/health/diseases/21490-enlarged-heart-cardiomegaly

**Chapter Thirteen:**

http://www.journals.elsevierhealth.com/periodicals/ymmt/article/PIIS0161475400901088/abstract

http://erbfamilyhyperbaric.com

https://spinalresearch.com.au/stress-brain-body-connection/

https://www.ncbi.nlm.nih.gov/pubmed/17615391

https://www.sharecare.com/health/digestive-health/how-brain-digestive-system-together

https://www.ncbi.nlm.nih.gov/books/NBK279994/

https://www.pharmaceutical-technology.com/features/biggest-pharma-ceutical-lawsuits/?fbclid=IwAR1SNeeLPYsXJZTKa3n1cqIla1s3wQeT-09m5avO-3yJQNxOXjR7ruKdNGtY

Korr 1979

J. BONE JOINT SURG. AM 1981 JUN;63(5):702-12

Web MD (Supplements)

https://spinalresearch.com.au/stress-brain-body-connection/

https://www.ncbi.nlm.nih.gov/pubmed/17615391

https://www.merckmanuals.com/home/brain,-spinal-cord,-and-nerve-disorders/biology-of-the-nervous-system/spinal-cord

https://www.healthline.com/human-body-maps/kidney#nephrons)

https://spinalresearch.com.au/stress-brain-body-connection/

https://www.ncbi.nlm.nih.gov/books/NBK10877/

https://www.mindbodygreen.com/0-14560/10-reasons-why-stress-is-the-most-dangerous-toxin-in-your-life.html

https://pdfs.semanticscholar.org/a4af/f1e3f1a555e-2868a306b70123525dd5f713c.pdf

**http://pathwaystofamilywellness.org/Wellness-Lifestyle/the-stress-paradox.html**

https://pdfs.semanticscholar.org/a4af/f1e3f1a555e-2868a306b70123525dd5f713c.pdf

https://www.health.harvard.edu/blog/nutritional-psychiatry-your-brain-on-food-201511168626

https://www.ncbi.nlm.nih.gov/pmc/articles/PMC3605358/

https://www.healthline.com/health/stomach-massage

https://www.healthline.com/nutrition/10-benefits-of-exercise#section9

https://www.sciencedirect.com/science/article/pii/
S1744388117304693?via%3Dihub

https://www.ncbi.nlm.nih.gov/pmc/articles/PMC3755035/

http://erbfamilyhyperbaric.com

https://psychcentral.com/lib/understanding-recognizing-stress/

https://www.mayoclinic.org/healthy-lifestyle/stress-management/
in-depth/stress/art-20046037

https://www.verywellmind.com/
what-is-the-fight-or-flight-response-2795194

**https://www.webmd.com/balance/stress-management/
stress-symptoms-effects_of-stress-on-the-body#2_**

**https://www.healthline.com/health/emotional-symptoms-of-stress**

https://www.drz.org/asp/NL/NL_Exercise_Oxygen_Cancer_OL_10.18.12.
htm

https://erbfamilythermography.com

**https://www.themindfulnessclinic.ca/high-intensity-interval-train-
ing-hiit-for-anxiety-depression-and-fitness/**

https://www.youtube.com/watch?v=dw_4hTK1_ek

http://erbfamilyhyperbaric.com

https://www.defendershield.com/
emf-immune-system-affects-disease-chronic-illness

https://www.greenmedinfo.com/blog/groundbreak-
ing-study-shows-shielding-emf-improves-autoimmune-disease1